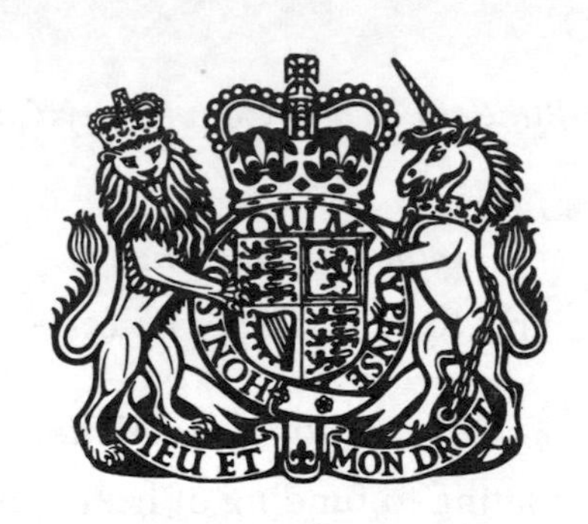

National Health Service and Community Care Act 1990

CHAPTER 19

ARRANGEMENT OF SECTIONS

PART I

THE NATIONAL HEALTH SERVICE: ENGLAND AND WALES

Local management

PART III

COMMUNITY CARE: ENGLAND AND WALES

Provision of accommodation and welfare services

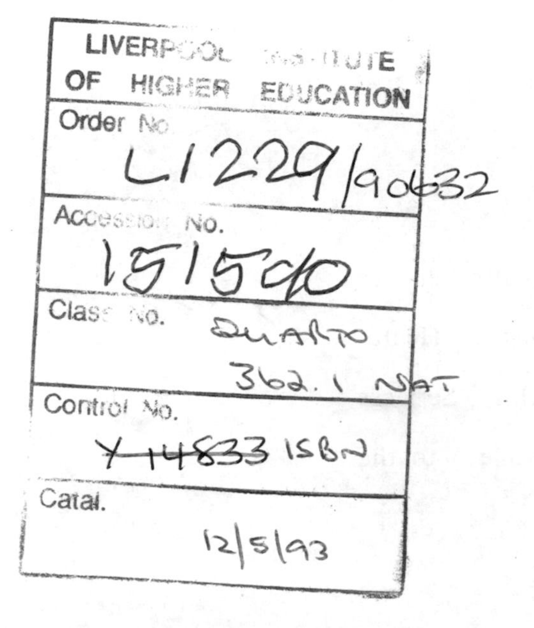

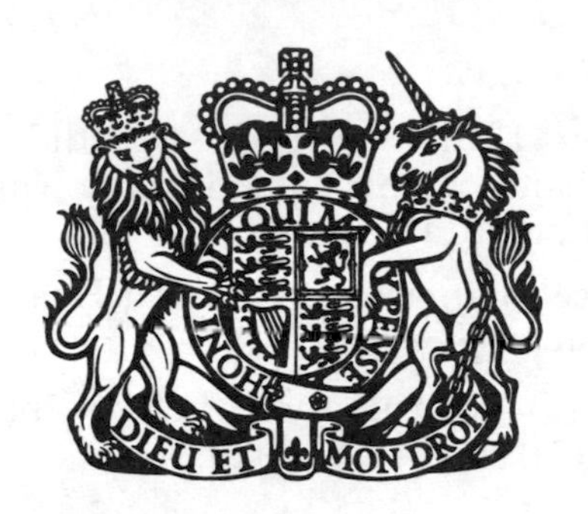

National Health Service and Community Care Act 1990

1990 CHAPTER 19

An Act to make further provision about health authorities and other bodies constituted in accordance with the National Health Service Act 1977; to provide for the establishment of National Health Service trusts; to make further provision about the financing of the practices of medical practitioners; to amend Part VII of the Local Government (Scotland) Act 1973 and Part III of the Local Government Finance Act 1982; to amend the National Health Service Act 1977 and the National Health Service (Scotland) Act 1978; to amend Part VIII of the Mental Health (Scotland) Act 1984; to make further provision concerning the provision of accommodation and other welfare services by local authorities and the powers of the Secretary of State as respects the social services functions of such authorities; to make provision for and in connection with the establishment of a Clinical Standards Advisory Group; to repeal the Health Services Act 1976; and for connected purposes.

[29th June 1990]

BE IT ENACTED by the Queen's most Excellent Majesty, by and with the advice and consent of the Lords Spiritual and Temporal, and Commons, in this present Parliament assembled, and by the authority of the same, as follows:—

PART I

THE NATIONAL HEALTH SERVICE: ENGLAND AND WALES

Local management

Regional and District Health Authorities. 1977 c. 49.

1.—(1) In the National Health Service Act 1977 (in this Part of this Act referred to as "the principal Act"), in section 8 (Regional and District Health Authorities etc.)—

PART I

(a) in subsection (1) for the words "Schedule 5 to this Act" there shall bc substituted "Schedule 1 to the National Health Service and Community Care Act 1990";

(b) any reference to an area or an Area Health Authority shall be omitted; and

(c) subsection (5) (consultation before making orders under subsection (2)) shall be omitted.

(2) Part I of Schedule 1 to this Act shall have effect in place of Part I of Schedule 5 to the principal Act (membership of health authorities etc.).

(3) Part III of Schedule 5 to the principal Act (supplementary provisions as to authorities) shall be amended in accordance with Part III of Schedule 1 to this Act.

(4) Subject to subsection (5) below, at the end of the day appointed for the coming into force of this subsection,—

(a) any person who became a member of a Regional or District Health Authority under Part I of Schedule 5 to the principal Act shall cease to be such a member; and

(b) any person who, by virtue of an order under section 11 of the principal Act, became a member of a special health authority which is a relevant authority for the purposes of paragraph 9(1) of Schedule 5 to that Act (as amended by Part III of Schedule 1 to this Act) shall cease to be such a member.

(5) Subsection (4) above does not apply to a person holding office as chairman of a Regional, District or Special Health Authority.

Family Health Services Authorities.

2.—(1) On and after the day appointed for the coming into force of this subsection—

(a) each existing Family Practitioner Committee shall be known as a Family Health Services Authority; and

(b) any reference in any enactment to a Family Practitioner Committee shall be construed as a reference to a Family Health Services Authority;

and the generality of this subsection is not affected by any express amendment made by this Act.

(2) In subsection (1) above "enactment" means—

(a) an enactment passed before the day appointed for the coming into force of subsection (1) above; and

(b) an enactment comprised in subordinate legislation made before that day.

(3) In section 10 of the principal Act (Family Health Services Authorities)—

(a) for the words "Schedule 5 to this Act" there shall be substituted "Schedule 1 to the National Health Service and Community Care Act 1990"; and

(b) subsection (7) (consultation before making orders under subsection (4)) shall be omitted.

(4) Part II of Schedule 1 to this Act shall have effect in place of Part II of Schedule 5 to the principal Act (membership of Family Practitioner Committees).

(5) At the end of the day appointed for the coming into force of this subsection, any person who became a member of a Family Practitioner Committee under Part II of Schedule 5 to the principal Act (including a person holding office as chairman of such a committee) shall cease to be a member and, accordingly, in the case of a chairman, shall also cease to be chairman.

(6) Nothing in this section shall cause a Family Health Services Authority to be included in the expression "health authority", as defined in the principal Act.

Primary and other functions of health authorities etc. and exercise of functions.

3.—(1) Any reference in this Act to the primary functions of a Regional, District or Special Health Authority is a reference to those functions for the time being exercisable by the authority by virtue of directions under section 11, section 13 or section 14 of the principal Act; and any reference in this Act to the primary functions of a Family Health Services Authority is a reference to the functions for the time being exercisable by the authority by virtue of this Act or section 15 of the principal Act.

(2) In addition to carrying out its primary functions, a Regional, District or Special Health Authority or a Family Health Services Authority may, as the provider, enter into an NHS contract (as defined in section 4 below) under which the goods or services to be provided are of the same description as goods or services which the authority already provides or could provide for the purposes of carrying out its primary functions.

(3) In section 16 of the principal Act (exercise of functions), in subsection (1) for the words from "an Area", in the first place where they occur, to "Health Authority" in the second place where those words occur, there shall be substituted "a Regional or District Health Authority, or exercisable by a Regional or District Health Authority by virtue of any prescribed provision of this or any other Act, or exercisable by a Family Health Services Authority under Part I of the National Health Service and Community Care Act 1990".

(4) In section 17 of the principal Act (directions as to exercise of functions), in subsection (1) after the words "sections 13 to 16 above" there shall be inserted "and may also give directions with respect to the exercise by health authorities or Family Health Services Authorities of functions under the National Health Service and Community Care Act 1990".

(5) Nothing in this section or in the principal Act affects the power of a Regional, District or Special Health Authority at any time to provide goods or services under the principal Act for the benefit of an individual where—

(a) the provision of those goods or services is neither within the primary functions of the authority nor carried out pursuant to an NHS contract; but

PART I

(b) the condition of the individual is such that he needs those goods or services and, having regard to his condition, it is not practicable before providing them to enter into an NHS contract for their provision.

(6) In any case where—

(a) a Regional, District or Special Health Authority provides goods or services for the benefit of an individual as mentioned in subsection (5) above, and

(b) the provision of those goods or services is within the primary functions of another health authority or is a function of a health board,

the authority providing the goods or services shall be remunerated in respect of that provision by that other health authority or health board.

(7) The rate of any remuneration payable by virtue of subsection (6) above shall be calculated in such manner or on such basis as may be determined by the Secretary of State.

(8) In any case where—

(a) a Regional, District or Special Health Authority provides goods or services for the benefit of an individual, and

(b) the provision of those goods or services is not pursuant to an NHS contract, and

(c) the individual is resident outside the United Kingdom and is of a description (being a description associating the individual with another country) specified for the purposes of this subsection by a direction made by the Secretary of State,

the authority shall be remunerated by the Secretary of State in respect of the provision of the goods or services in question at such rate or rates as he considers appropriate.

NHS contracts.

4.—(1) In this Act the expression "NHS contract" means an arrangement under which one health service body ("the acquirer") arranges for the provision to it by another health service body ("the provider") of goods or services which it reasonably requires for the purposes of its functions.

(2) In this section "health service body" means any of the following, namely,—

(a) a health authority;

(b) a health board;

(c) the Common Services Agency for the Scottish Health Service;

(d) a Family Health Services Authority;

(e) an NHS trust;

(f) a recognised fund-holding practice;

(g) the Dental Practice Board or the Scottish Dental Practice Board;

(h) the Public Health Laboratory Service Board; and

(i) the Secretary of State.

(3) Whether or not an arrangement which constitutes an NHS contract would, apart from this subsection, be a contract in law, it shall not be regarded for any purpose as giving rise to contractual rights or liabilities, but if any dispute arises with respect to such an arrangement, either party may refer the matter to the Secretary of State for determination under the following provisions of this section.

(4) If, in the course of negotiations intending to lead to an arrangement which will be an NHS contract, it appears to a health service body—

(a) that the terms proposed by another health service body are unfair by reason that the other is seeking to take advantage of its position as the only, or the only practicable, provider of the goods or services concerned or by reason of any other unequal bargaining position as between the prospective parties to the proposed arrangement, or

(b) that for any other reason arising out of the relative bargaining position of the prospective parties any of the terms of the proposed arrangement cannot be agreed,

that health service body may refer the terms of the proposed arrangement to the Secretary of State for determination under the following provisions of this section.

(5) Where a reference is made to the Secretary of State under subsection (3) or subsection (4) above, the Secretary of State may determine the matter himself or, if he considers it appropriate, appoint a person to consider and determine it in accordance with regulations.

(6) By his determination of a reference under subsection (4) above, the Secretary of State or, as the case may be, the person appointed under subsection (5) above may specify terms to be included in the proposed arrangement and may direct that it be proceeded with; and it shall be the duty of the prospective parties to the proposed arrangement to comply with any such directions.

(7) A determination of a reference under subsection (3) above may contain such directions (including directions as to payment) as the Secretary of State or, as the case may be, the person appointed under subsection (5) above considers appropriate to resolve the matter in dispute; and it shall be the duty of the parties to the NHS contract in question to comply with any such directions.

(8) Without prejudice to the generality of his powers on a reference under subsection (3) above, the Secretary of State or, as the case may be, the person appointed under subsection (5) above may by his determination in relation to an arrangement constituting an NHS contract vary the terms of the arrangement or bring it to an end; and where an arrangement is so varied or brought to an end—

(a) subject to paragraph (b) below, the variation or termination shall be treated as being effected by agreement between the parties; and

(b) the directions included in the determination by virtue of subsection (7) above may contain such provisions as the Secretary of State or, as the case may be, the person appointed under subsection (5) above considers appropriate in order satisfactorily to give effect to the variation or to bring the arrangement to an end.

PART I

(9) In subsection (2) above "NHS trust" includes—

1978 c. 29.

(a) such a trust established under the National Health Service (Scotland) Act 1978; and

(b) a body established in Northern Ireland and specified by an order made by statutory instrument by the Secretary of State as equivalent to an NHS trust established under this Part of this Act.

National Health Service trusts

NHS trusts.

5.—(1) Subject to subsection (2) or, as the case may be, subsection (3) below the Secretary of State may by order establish bodies, to be known as National Health Service trusts (in this Act referred to as NHS trusts),—

(a) to assume responsibility, in accordance with this Act, for the ownership and management of hospitals or other establishments or facilities which were previously managed or provided by Regional, District or Special Health Authorities; or

(b) to provide and manage hospitals or other establishments or facilities.

(2) In any case where the Secretary of State is considering whether to make an order under subsection (1) above establishing an NHS trust and the hospital, establishment or facility concerned is or is to be situated in England, he shall direct the relevant Regional Health Authority to consult, with respect to the proposal to establish the trust,—

(a) the relevant Community Health Council and such other persons or bodies as may be specified in the direction; and

(b) such other persons or bodies as the Authority considers appropriate;

and, within such period (if any) as the Secretary of State may determine, the relevant Regional Health Authority shall report the results of those consultations to the Secretary of State.

(3) In any case where the Secretary of State is considering whether to make an order under subsection (1) above establishing an NHS trust and the hospital, establishment or facility concerned is or is to be situated in Wales, he shall consult the relevant Community Health Council and such other persons and bodies as he considers appropriate.

(4) In subsections (2) and (3) above—

(a) any reference to the relevant Regional Health Authority is a reference to that Authority in whose region the hospital, establishment or other facility concerned is, or is to be, situated; and

(b) any reference to the relevant Community Health Council is a reference to the Council for the district, or part of the district, in which that hospital, establishment or other facility is, or is to be, situated.

(5) Every NHS trust—

(a) shall be a body corporate having a board of directors consisting of a chairman appointed by the Secretary of State and, subject to paragraph 5(2) of Schedule 2 to this Act, executive and non-executive directors (that is to say, directors who, subject to subsection (7) below, respectively are and are not employees of the trust); and

(b) shall have the functions conferred on it by an order under subsection (1) above and by Schedule 2 to this Act.

(6) The functions specified in an order under subsection (1) above shall include such functions as the Secretary of State considers appropriate in relation to the provision of services by the trust for one or more health authorities.

(7) The Secretary of State may by regulations make general provision with respect to—

(a) the qualifications for and the tenure of office of the chairman and directors of an NHS trust (including the circumstances in which they shall cease to hold, or may be removed from, office or may be suspended from performing the functions of the office);

(b) the persons by whom the directors and any of the officers are to be appointed and the manner of their appointment;

(c) the maximum and minimum numbers of the directors;

(d) the circumstances in which a person who is not an employee of the trust is nevertheless, on appointment as a director, to be regarded as an executive rather than a non-executive director;

(e) the proceedings of the trust (including the validation of proceedings in the event of a vacancy or defect in appointment); and

(f) the appointment, constitution and exercise of functions by committees and sub-committees of the trust (whether or not consisting of or including any members of the board) and, without prejudice to the generality of the power, any such regulations, may make provision to deal with cases where the post of any officer of an NHS trust is held jointly by two or more persons or where the functions of such an officer are in any other way performed by more than one person.

(8) Part I of Schedule 2 to this Act shall have effect with respect to orders under subsection (1) above; Part II of that Schedule shall have effect, subject to subsection (9) below, with respect to the general duties and the powers and status of NHS trusts; the supplementary provisions of Part III of that Schedule shall have effect; and Part IV of that Schedule shall have effect with respect to the dissolution of NHS trusts.

(9) The specific powers conferred by paragraphs 14 and 15 in Part II of Schedule 2 to this Act may be exercised only to the extent that—

(a) the exercise will not interfere with the duties of the trust to comply with directions under paragraph 6 of that Schedule; and

(b) the exercise will not to any significant extent interfere with the performance by the trust of its obligations under any NHS contract or any obligations imposed by an order under subsection (1) above.

PART I

(10) The Secretary of State may by order made by statutory instrument confer on NHS trusts specific powers additional to those contained in paragraphs 10 to 15 of Schedule 2 to this Act.

Transfer of staff to NHS trusts.

6.—(1) Subject to subsection (5) below, this section applies to any person who, immediately before an NHS trust's operational date—

(a) is employed by a health authority to work solely at, or for the purposes of, a hospital or other establishment or facility which is to become the responsibility of the trust; or

(b) is employed by a health authority to work at, or for the purposes of, such a hospital, establishment or facility and is designated for the purposes of this section by a scheme made by the health authority specified as mentioned in paragraph 3(1)(f) of Schedule 2 to this Act.

(2) A scheme under this section shall not have effect unless approved by the Secretary of State.

(3) Subject to section 7 below, the contract of employment between a person to whom this section applies and the health authority by whom he is employed shall have effect from the operational date as if originally made between him and the NHS trust.

(4) Without prejudice to subsection (3) above—

(a) all the health authority's rights, powers, duties and liabilities under or in connection with a contract to which that subsection applies shall by virtue of this section be transferred to the NHS trust on its operational date; and

(b) anything done before that date by or in relation to the health authority in respect of that contract or the employee shall be deemed from that date to have been done by or in relation to the NHS trust.

(5) In any case where—

(a) an order under section 5(1) above provides for the establishment of an NHS trust with effect from a date earlier than the operational date of the trust, and

(b) on or after that earlier date but before its operational date the NHS trust makes an offer of employment by the trust to a person who at that time is employed by a health authority to work (whether solely or otherwise) at, or for the purposes of, the hospital or other establishment or facility which is to become the responsibility of the trust, and

(c) as a result of the acceptance of the offer, the person to whom it was made becomes an employee of the NHS trust,

subsections (3) and (4) above shall have effect in relation to that person's contract of employment as if he were a person to whom this section applies and any reference in those subsections to the operational date of the trust were a reference to the date on which he takes up employment with the trust.

PART I

(6) Subsections (3) and (4) above are without prejudice to any right of an employee to terminate his contract of employment if a substantial change is made to his detriment in his working conditions; but no such right shall arise by reason only of the change in employer effected by this section.

(7) A scheme under this section may designate a person either individually or as a member of a class or description of employees.

Supplementary provisions as to transfer of staff.

7.—(1) In the case of a person who falls within section 6(1)(b) above, a scheme under that section may provide that, with effect from the NHS trust's operational date, his contract of employment (in this section referred to as "his original contract") shall be treated in accordance with the scheme as divided so as to constitute—

(a) a contract of employment with the NHS trust; and

(b) a contract of employment with the health authority by whom he was employed before that date (in this section referred to as "the transferor authority").

(2) Where a scheme makes provision as mentioned in subsection (1) above,—

(a) the scheme shall secure that the benefits to the employee under the two contracts referred to in that subsection, when taken together, are not less favourable than the benefits under his original contract;

(b) section 6 above shall apply in relation to the contract referred to in subsection (1)(a) above as if it were a contract transferred under that section from the transferor authority to the NHS trust;

(c) so far as necessary to preserve any rights and obligations, the contract referred to in subsection (1)(b) above shall be regarded as a continuation of the employee's original contract; and

(d) for the purposes of section 146 of and Schedule 13 to the Employment Protection (Consolidation) Act 1978, the number of hours normally worked, or, as the case may be, the hours for which the employee is employed in any week under either of those contracts shall be taken to be the total of the hours normally worked or, as the case may be, for which he is employed under the two contracts taken together.

1978 c. 44.

(3) Where, as a result of the provisions of section 6 above, by virtue of his employment during any period after the operational date of the NHS trust,—

(a) an employee has contractual rights against an NHS trust to benefits in the event of his redundancy, and

(b) he also has statutory rights against the trust under Part VI of the Employment Protection (Consolidation) Act 1978 (redundancy payments),

any benefits provided to him by virtue of the contractual rights referred to in paragraph (a) above shall be taken as satisfying his entitlement to benefits under the said Part VI.

PART I

Transfer of property, rights and liabilities to NHS trust.

8.—(1) The Secretary of State may by order transfer or provide for the transfer to an NHS trust, with effect from such date as may be specified in the order, of such of the property, rights and liabilities of a health authority or of the Secretary of State as, in his opinion, need to be transferred to the trust for the purpose of enabling it to carry out its functions.

(2) An order under this section may create or impose such new rights or liabilities in respect of what is transferred or what is retained by a health authority or the Secretary of State as appear to him to be necessary or expedient.

(3) Nothing in this section affects the power of the Secretary of State or any power of a health authority to transfer property, rights or liabilities to an NHS trust otherwise than under subsection (1) above.

(4) Stamp duty shall not be chargeable in respect of any transfer to an NHS trust effected by or by virtue of an order under this section.

(5) Where an order under this section provides for the transfer—

(a) of land held on lease from a third party, that is to say, a person other than the Secretary of State or a health authority, or

(b) of any other asset leased or hired from a third party or in which a third party has an interest,

the transfer shall be binding on the third party notwithstanding that, apart from this subsection, it would have required his consent or concurrence.

(6) Any property, rights and liabilities which are to be transferred to an NHS trust shall be identified by agreement between the trust and a health authority or, in default of agreement, by direction of the Secretary of State.

(7) Where, for the purpose of a transfer pursuant to an order under this section, it becomes necessary to apportion any property, rights or liabilities, the order may contain such provisions as appear to the Secretary of State to be appropriate for the purpose; and where any such property or rights fall within subsection (5) above, the order shall contain such provisions as appear to the Secretary of State to be appropriate to safeguard the interests of third parties, including, where appropriate, provision for the payment of compensation of an amount to be determined in accordance with the order.

(8) In the case of any transfer made by or pursuant to an order under this section, a certificate issued by the Secretary of State that any property specified in the certificate or any such interest in or right over any such property as may be so specified, or any right or liability so specified, is vested in the NHS trust specified in the order shall be conclusive evidence of that fact for all purposes.

(9) Without prejudice to subsection (4) of section 126 of the principal Act, an order under this section may include provision for matters to be settled by arbitration by a person determined in accordance with the order.

Originating capital debt of, and other financial provisions relating to NHS trusts.

9.—(1) Each NHS trust shall have an originating capital debt of an amount specified in an order made by the Secretary of State, being an amount representing, subject to subsection (2) below, the excess of the valuation of the assets which, on or in connection with the establishment

PART I

of the trust, are or are to be transferred to it (whether before, on or after its operational date) over the amounts of the liabilities which are or are to be so transferred.

(2) In determining the originating capital debt of an NHS trust, there shall be left out of account such assets or, as the case may be, liabilities as are, or are of a class, determined for the purposes of this section by the Secretary of State, with the consent of the Treasury.

(3) An NHS trust's originating capital debt shall be deemed to have been issued out of moneys provided by Parliament and shall constitute an asset of the Consolidated Fund.

(4) In accordance with an order under subsection (1) above, an NHS trust's originating capital debt shall be divided between—

(a) a loan on which interest shall be paid at such variable or fixed rates and at such times as the Treasury may determine; and

(b) public dividend capital.

(5) The loan specified in subsection (4)(a) above is in this Part of this Act referred to as an NHS trust's "initial loan" and a rate of interest on the initial loan shall be determined as if section 5 of the National Loans Act 1968 had effect in respect of it and subsections (5) to (5B) of that section shall apply accordingly.

1968. c. 13.

(6) Subject to subsections (4)(a) and (5) above, the terms of the initial loan shall be such as the Secretary of State, with the consent of the Treasury, may determine; and, in the event of the early repayment of the initial loan, the terms may require the payment of a premium or allow a discount.

(7) With the consent of the Treasury, the Secretary of State may determine the terms on which any public dividend capital forming part of an NHS trust's originating capital debt is to be treated as having been issued, and, in particular, may determine the dividend which is to be payable at any time on any public dividend capital.

(8) An order under subsection (1) above shall be made—

(a) with the consent of the Treasury; and

(b) by statutory instrument.

(9) Schedule 3 to this Act shall have effect with respect to—

(a) borrowing by NHS trusts;

(b) the limits on their indebtedness;

(c) the payment of additional public dividend capital to them; and

(d) the application of any surplus funds of NHS trusts.

Financial obligations of NHS trusts.

10.—(1) Every NHS trust shall ensure that its revenue is not less than sufficient, taking one financial year with another, to meet outgoings properly chargeable to revenue account.

(2) It shall be the duty of every NHS trust to achieve such financial objectives as may from time to time be set by the Secretary of State with the consent of the Treasury and as are applicable to it; and any such objectives may be made applicable to NHS trusts generally, or to a particular NHS trust or to NHS trusts of a particular description.

PART I

Trust funds and trustees for NHS trusts.

11.—(1) The Secretary of State may by order made by statutory instrument provide for the appointment of trustees for an NHS trust; and any trustees so appointed shall have power to accept, hold and administer any property on trust for the general or any specific purposes of the NHS trust (including the purposes of any specific hospital or other establishment or facility which is owned and managed by the trust) or for all or any purposes relating to the health service.

(2) An order under subsection (1) above may—

(a) make provision as to the persons by whom trustees are to be appointed and generally as to the method of their appointment;

(b) make any appointment subject to such conditions as may be specified in the order (including conditions requiring the consent of the Secretary of State);

(c) make provision as to the number of trustees to be appointed, including provision under which that number may from time to time be determined by the Secretary of State after consultation with such persons as he considers appropriate; and

(d) make provision with respect to the term of office of any trustee and his removal from office.

(3) Where, under subsection (1) above, trustees have been appointed for an NHS trust, the Secretary of State may by order made by statutory instrument provide for the transfer of any trust property from the NHS trust to the trustees so appointed.

(4) In section 91 of the principal Act (private trusts for hospitals) in subsection (3) (definition of "the appropriate hospital authority") after paragraph (a) there shall be inserted the following paragraphs—

"(aa) where the hospital is owned and managed by an NHS trust and trustees have been appointed for the NHS trust, those trustees;

(ab) where the hospital is owned and managed by an NHS trust and neither paragraph (a) nor paragraph (aa) above applies, the NHS trust;".

(5) In section 92 of the principal Act (further transfers of trust property)—

(a) in subsection (1) after the word "hospital" there shall be inserted "or other establishment or facility" and for the words "or special trustees", in each place where they occur, there shall be substituted "NHS trust, special trustees or trustees for an NHS trust";

(b) in subsections (2) to (4), after the word "authorities", in each place where it occurs, there shall be inserted "or NHS trusts";

(c) in subsection (2) after the word "authority", there shall be inserted "or NHS trust"; and

(d) at the end of the section there shall be added the following subsection—

"(6) If it appears to the Secretary of State at any time that—

(a) the functions of any special trustees should be discharged by the trustees for an NHS trust, or

(b) the functions of the trustees for an NHS trust should be discharged by special trustees,

then, whether or not there has been any such change as is mentioned in subsection (1) above, he may, after consulting the special trustees and the trustees for the NHS trust, by order provide for the transfer of all trust property from or to the special trustees to or from the trustees for the NHS trust."

(6) In section 96 of the principal Act (trusts: supplementary provisions)—

(a) any reference to sections 90 to 95 of the principal Act includes a reference to subsections (1) to (3) above; and

(b) after subsection (1) there shall be inserted the following subsection—

"(1A) Where any transfer of property by virtue of those sections is of, or includes,—

(a) land held on lease from a third party, that is to say, a person other than the Secretary of State or a health authority, or

(b) any other asset leased or hired from a third party or in which a third party has an interest,

the transfer shall be binding on the third party notwithstanding that, apart from this subsection, it would have required his consent or concurrence."

(7) In section 98(1) of the principal Act (accounts and audit) after paragraph (d) there shall be inserted—

"(dd) any trustees for an NHS trust appointed in pursuance of section 11 of the National Health Service and Community Care Act 1990; and".

Family Health Services Authorities

Functions of Family Health Services Authorities.

12.—(1) In section 15 of the principal Act (duty of Family Health Services Authority)—

(a) in subsection (1), after the word "regulations" there shall be inserted "and subject to any directions from the relevant Regional Health Authority";

(b) in paragraph (b) of that subsection, after the words "perform such" there shall be inserted "management and"; and

(c) at the end of that subsection there shall be inserted the following subsections—

"(1A) In relation to a Family Health Services Authority for a locality in England, any reference in this Act or the National Health Service and Community Care Act 1990 to the relevant Regional Health Authority is a reference to that Authority in whose region lies the whole or the greater part of the Authority's locality.

(1B) In relation to a medical practitioner, any reference in this Act or the National Health Service and Community Care Act 1990 to the relevant Family Health Services Authority shall be construed as follows,—

PART I

(a) if he practices in partnership with other medical practitioners, the relevant Authority is that Authority on whose medical list the members of the practice are included and, if some are included on one Authority's medical list and some on another's or if any of the members is included in the medical lists of two or more Authorities, the relevant Authority is that Authority in whose locality resides the largest number of individuals who are on the lists of patients of the members of the practice; and

(b) in any other case, the relevant Authority is that Authority on whose medical list he is included and, if there is more than one, that one of them in whose locality resides the largest number of individuals who are on his list of patients."

(2) In section 17 of the principal Act (directions as to exercise of functions), in subsection (1) before the words "by a District Health Authority", there shall be inserted "(a)" and at the end of the subsection there shall be added "and

(b) by a Family Health Services Authority in relation to which it is the relevant Regional Health Authority, of any functions exercisable by the Family Health Services Authority by virtue of section 15 above or the National Health Service and Community Care Act 1990."

(3) In section 42 of the principal Act (regulations as to pharmaceutical services), in subsection (3)—

(a) in paragraph (d) for the words following "approved by" there shall be substituted "reference to prescribed criteria by the Family Health Services Authority in whose locality those premises are situated; and"; and

(b) in paragraph (e) for the words "the prescribed body" there shall be substituted "that Family Health Services Authority".

(4) In section 44 of the principal Act (recognition by Secretary of State of certain local committees), in subsection (1)—

(a) for the words from "the Secretary of State" to "is representative" there shall be substituted "a Family Health Services Authority is satisfied that a committee formed for its locality is representative"; and

(b) for the word "he" there shall be substituted "the Family Health Services Authority";

and in subsection (2) of that section, for the words "Secretary of State's approval" there shall be substituted "approval of the Family Health Services Authority".

(5) Section 55 of the principal Act (reference of certain disputes affecting Family Practitioner Committees to the Secretary of State) shall cease to have effect.

Financial duties in relation to Family Health Services Authorities.

13.—(1) Section 97A of the principal Act (financial duties of health authorities) shall be amended in accordance with subsections (2) to (4) below.

(2) In subsection (1) for the words from "the expenditure attributable" to the end of the subsection there shall be substituted—

"(a) the expenditure attributable to the performance by the Regional Health Authority of its functions in that year, and

(b) the expenditure attributable to the performance by the District Health Authorities whose districts are in the region of their functions in that year, and

(c) the expenditure attributable to the performance by each Family Health Services Authority in relation to which the Regional Health Authority is the relevant Regional Health Authority of the Family Health Services Authority's functions in that year, other than expenditure falling within section 97(1)(aa) above,

does not exceed the aggregate of—

(i) the amounts allotted to the Regional Health Authority for that year under section 97(1)(a) above;

(ii) any other sums received under this Act, other than under section 97(1)(aa) above, in that year by the Regional Health Authority or by the District Health Authorities or Family Health Services Authorities concerned; and

(iii) any sums received otherwise than under this Act in that year by any of those Authorities for the purpose of enabling them to defray any such expenditure".

(3) In subsection (2)—

(a) for the words "Area Health Authority and every District Health Authority" there shall be substituted "District Health Authority and every Family Health Services Authority";

(b) in paragraph (a) of that subsection after the word "above" there shall be inserted "other than section 97(1)(aa)".

(4) In subsection (4) after the words "health authority" there shall be inserted "or Family Health Services Authority".

(5) In section 97B of the principal Act, in subsection (1)—

(a) for the words "Family Practitioner Committee" there shall be substituted "Family Health Services Authority whose locality is in Wales"; and

(b) at the end there shall be added the words "and any reference in subsections (2) and (4) below to a Family Health Services Authority is a reference to an Authority whose locality is in Wales".

Fund-holding practices

Recognition of fund-holding practices of doctors.

14.—(1) Any one or more medical practitioners who are providing general medical services in accordance with arrangements under section 29 of the principal Act may apply to the relevant Regional Health Authority for recognition as a fund-holding practice.

PART I

(2) The relevant Regional Health Authority shall not grant recognition as a fund-holding practice unless the medical practitioner or, as the case may be, each of the medical practitioners concerned fulfils such conditions as may be prescribed.

(3) Subject to subsection (4) below, in relation to a medical practitioner, any reference in this Part of this Act to the relevant Regional Health Authority is a reference to that Authority which, in relation to the practitioner's relevant Family Health Services Authority, is the relevant Regional Health Authority.

(4) Where two or more medical practitioners wish to make an application under subsection (1) above and, apart from this subsection, the relevant Family Health Services Authority in respect of one or more of them would be different from that in respect of the other or others, then, for the purposes of this section and any other provisions relating to fund-holding practices, the relevant Family Health Services Authority for each of them shall be determined as if they were all practising in a single partnership.

(5) In the application of this section to any medical practitioner whose relevant Family Health Services Authority has a locality in Wales, for any reference to the relevant Regional Health Authority there shall be substituted a reference to the Secretary of State.

(6) Regulations may make provision with respect to—

(a) the making of applications under subsection (1) above;

(b) the granting and refusal of recognition as a fund-holding practice;

(c) the conditions to be fulfilled for obtaining and continuing to be entitled to such recognition;

(d) appeals against any refusal of such recognition by a Regional Health Authority;

(e) withdrawing from, or becoming a member of, an existing recognised fund-holding practice;

(f) the continuity or otherwise of a recognised fund-holding practice in the event of the death or withdrawal of a member or the addition of a new member; and

(g) the operation of this section in a case where one or more of the medical practitioners wishing to make an application under subsection (1) above is also on the medical list of a health board;

and regulations making the provision referred to in paragraph (g) above may make such modifications of the preceding provisions of this section as the Secretary of State considers appropriate.

Payments to recognised fund-holding practices.

15.—(1) In respect of each financial year, every Regional Health Authority shall be liable to pay to the members of each recognised fund-holding practice in relation to which it is the relevant Regional Health Authority a sum determined in such manner and by reference to such factors as the Secretary of State may direct (in this section referred to as an "allotted sum").

(2) In respect of each financial year, the Secretary of State shall be liable to pay to the members of each recognised fund-holding practice whose relevant Family Health Services Authority has a locality in Wales a sum determined in such manner and by reference to such factors as the Secretary of State may direct (in this section referred to as an "allotted sum").

(3) The liability to pay an allotted sum under subsection (1) or subsection (2) above may be discharged, in whole or in part, in either of the following ways—

(a) by making payments on account of the allotted sum at such times and in such manner as the Secretary of State may direct; and

(b) by discharging liabilities of the members of the practice to any other person (including, in particular, liabilities under NHS contracts);

and any reference in the following provisions of this Part of this Act to payment of or of a part of an allotted sum includes a reference to the discharge, in accordance with this subsection, of the whole or part of the liability to pay that sum.

(4) In any case where—

(a) a Regional Health Authority makes a payment of or of any part of an allotted sum to the members of a recognised fund-holding practice, and

(b) some of the individuals on the list of patients of any of the members of the practice reside in the region of another Regional Health Authority, or in Wales, or in the area of a Health Board,

the Authority making the payment shall be entitled to recover from that other Authority or, as the case may be, from the Secretary of State or that Health Board an amount equal to such portion of the payment as may be determined in accordance with directions given by the Secretary of State.

(5) In any case where—

(a) the Secretary of State makes a payment of or of any part of an allotted sum to the members of a recognised fund-holding practice, and

(b) some of the individuals on the list of patients of any of the members of the practice reside in the region of a Regional Health Authority,

the Secretary of State shall be entitled to recover from that Authority an amount equal to such portion of the payment as may be determined in accordance with directions given by the Secretary of State.

(6) The members of a recognised fund-holding practice may apply an allotted sum only for purposes specified in regulations under subsection (7) below.

(7) Regulations shall make provision with respect to the purposes for which allotted sums are to be or may be applied and may make provision generally with respect to the operation of recognised fund-holding practices in relation to allotted sums; and the regulations may, in particular,—

PART I

(a) require the members of a practice to pay to the relevant Regional Health Authority out of allotted sums paid to them an amount determined in accordance with the regulations as the basic cost of the drugs, medicines and listed appliances supplied pursuant to orders given by or on behalf of members of the practice;

(b) provide that the goods and services, other than general medical services, which may be purchased by or on behalf of the members of a practice out of allotted sums for the individuals on the lists of patients of the members of the practice shall be such as may be specified in a list approved for the purpose under the regulations; and

(c) impose a limit on the amount which may be spent out of an allotted sum on the provision of goods and services for any one individual, being a limit above which the cost of any goods and services for that individual in the financial year in question will fall to be met by the District Health Authority whose primary functions include the provision of goods and services (not necessarily the goods and services in question) to the individual concerned.

(8) In the application of subsection (7) above to the members of a practice whose relevant Family Health Services Authority has a locality in Wales, for the reference in paragraph (a) of that subsection to the relevant Regional Health Authority there shall be substituted a reference to the Secretary of State.

(9) In accordance with directions under section 17 of the principal Act, the relevant Family Health Services Authority shall monitor the expenditure of the members of a recognised fund-holding practice and may institute an audit and review in any case where the Authority consider it necessary to do so.

Renunciation and removal of recognition as a fund-holding practice and withholding of funds.

16.—(1) Regulations may make provision as to the circumstances in which the members of a recognised fund-holding practice may renounce that status and such regulations may, in particular, make provision as to—

(a) the notice to be given and the number of members of the practice by whom it is to be given;

(b) the procedure to be followed; and

(c) the consequences of such a renunciation.

(2) Regulations may make provision as to the circumstances in which and the grounds on which the relevant Regional Health Authority or, as the case may be, the Secretary of State may remove recognition from the members of a fund-holding practice,—

(a) with immediate effect; or

(b) with effect from the end of a particular financial year; or

(c) with effect from such other date as may be specified by the Regional Health Authority or, as the case may be, the Secretary of State.

(3) Where provision is made as mentioned in subsection (2) above, regulations shall make provision with respect to—

(a) the procedure for the removal of recognition;

(b) appeals against the removal of recognition by a Regional Health Authority; and

(c) the consequences of the removal of recognition.

(4) Without prejudice to the generality of the powers conferred by subsection (3) above, regulations making provision as mentioned in paragraph (c) of that subsection—

(a) may provide for the transfer of rights and obligations from the members of the fund-holding practice to one or more District Health Authorities determined in accordance with the regulations;

(b) may provide for the recovery of sums from the members of the practice; and

(c) may require the members of the practice to furnish such information as may reasonably be required by the Regional Health Authority or, as the case may be, the Secretary of State.

(5) The bringing of an appeal against the removal of recognition by a Regional Health Authority shall not be regarded as preserving the recognised status of the members of the fund-holding practice and, accordingly, subject to the outcome of the appeal, the relevant Regional Health Authority shall not be required, after the removal takes effect, to make any (or, as the case may be, any further) payment to the members of the practice of any part of the allotted sum for the financial year in question or, as the case may be, to determine and pay any allotted sum for a future financial year.

(6) Where any part of an allotted sum has been applied by the members of a recognised fund-holding practice (or any one or more of them) for purposes other than those specified in regulations under section 15(7) above, regulations may make provision for and in connection with the recovery by the relevant Regional Health Authority or, as the case may be, the Secretary of State of an amount equal to that part.

(7) Where provision is made as mentioned in subsection (6) above, regulations shall make provision with respect to appeals against the recovery of any amount by a Regional Health Authority.

Transfer of functions relating to recognised fund-holding practices.

17.—(1) If the Secretary of State by regulations so provides, such of the functions of a Regional Health Authority or, in Wales, the Secretary of State under sections 14 to 16 above as are specified in, or determined in accordance with, the regulations shall become functions of a Family Health Services Authority with effect from such date as may be prescribed.

(2) Regulations under this section shall make provision for determining the Family Health Services Authority which is to exercise any of the functions concerned in relation to the members of any existing recognised fund-holding practice and in relation to any medical practitioners wishing to apply for recognition.

(3) Without prejudice to the generality of section 126(4) of the principal Act, regulations under this section may make such incidental and consequential modifications of the principal Act and of sections 14 to 16 above as appear to the Secretary of State to be necessary or expedient in consequence of the transfer of functions effected by the regulations.

PART I

Indicative amounts

Indicative amounts for doctors' practices.

18.—(1) Subject to subsection (2) below, for each financial year, every Family Health Services Authority shall, by notice in writing given to each practice in relation to the members of which it is the relevant Family Health Services Authority, specify an amount of money (in this Act referred to as an "indicative amount") representing the basic price of the drugs, medicines and listed appliances which, in the opinion of the Authority, it is reasonable to expect will be supplied in that year pursuant to orders given by or on behalf of the members of that practice.

(2) Subsection (1) above does not apply with respect to a practice which is or forms part of a fund-holding practice recognised under section 14 above.

(3) For the purposes of this section, a "practice" means—

(a) a single medical practitioner who practises otherwise than in partnership; or

(b) any two or more medical practitioners who practise in partnership;

and any reference to the members of a practice shall be construed accordingly.

(4) The members of a practice shall seek to secure that, except with the consent of the relevant Family Health Services Authority or for good cause, the orders for drugs, medicines and listed appliances given by them or on their behalf are such that the basic price of the items supplied pursuant to those orders in any financial year does not exceed the indicative amount notified to the practice for that year under subsection (1) above.

(5) For the purpose of measuring the extent to which a practice is operating within the indicative amount notified to it under subsection (1) above for any financial year, a Family Health Services Authority shall set against that indicative amount an amount equal to the basic price of the drugs, medicines and listed appliances supplied in that year pursuant to orders given by or on behalf of members of the practice.

(6) For the purposes of this section, regulations may make provision as to the specification of, or means of calculating, the basic price of any drugs, medicines or listed appliances.

1978 c. 29.

(7) If, in the case of any practice, a member is on the medical list of a Health Board constituted under section 2 of the National Health Service (Scotland) Act 1978 (as well as on that of a Family Health Services Authority), any question whether this section applies in relation to the members of the practice shall be determined in accordance with regulations made by the Secretary of State; and any such regulations may modify the preceding provisions of this section in their application to such a practice.

Funding, audit and liabilities

Amendments relating to funding of health authorities etc.

19.—(1) Section 97 of the principal Act (means of meeting expenditure of health authorities out of public funds) shall be amended in accordance with this section.

(2) In subsection (1) (payments to health authorities etc. by the Secretary of State)—

(a) at the end of paragraph (a) there shall be added "including, in the case of a Regional Health Authority, its functions with respect to such expenditure of Family Health Services Authorities in relation to which it is the relevant Regional Health Authority as—

(i) is attributable to the reimbursement of expenses of persons providing services in pursuance of Part II of this Act and is of a description specified in the allotment, and

(ii) is attributable to the performance by the Family Health Services Authority of their functions in that year";

(b) after paragraph (a) there shall be inserted the following paragraph—

"(aa) to each Regional Health Authority sums equal to any such expenditure of Family Health Services Authorities in relation to which it is the relevant Regional Health Authority as is attributable to the remuneration of persons providing services in pursuance of Part II of this Act and is not of a description specified as mentioned in paragraph (a) above"; and

(c) in paragraph (b) for the words "Family Practitioner Committee" there shall be inserted "Family Health Services Authority whose locality is in Wales".

(3) In subsection (2) (payments by Regional Health Authorities) for the words following "each financial year" there shall be substituted—

"(a) to each District Health Authority whose district is included in the region sums not exceeding the amount allotted by the Regional Health Authority to the District Health Authority for that year towards meeting the expenditure attributable to the performance by the District Health Authority of their functions in that year; and

(b) to each Family Health Services Authority in relation to which it is the relevant Regional Health Authority—

(i) sums equal to the expenditure referred to in subsection (1)(aa) above; and

(ii) sums not exceeding the amount allotted by the Regional Health Authority to the Family Health Services Authority for that year towards meeting other expenditure attributable to the reimbursement of expenses of persons providing services in pursuance of Part II of this Act and to the performance by the Family Health Services Authority of their functions in that year."

(4) In subsection (3) (directions of Secretary of State)—

(a) after the word "directions" there shall be inserted "(a)";

(b) after the word "Regional" there shall be inserted "or Special" and for the words "Practitioner Committee" there shall be substituted "Health Services Authority whose locality is in Wales"; and

(c) at the end of the subsection there shall be added "and

PART I

(b) to a District Health Authority in England with respect to the payment of sums by them to the Regional Health Authority in respect of charges or other sums referable to the valuation or disposal of assets; and

(c) to a Regional Health Authority with respect to the application of sums received by them by virtue of paragraph (b) above or by virtue of section 15(7)(a) of the National Health Service and Community Care Act 1990."

(5) In subsection (4) (directions of Regional Health Authorities) for the words from "an Area Health Authority" onwards there shall be substituted "a District Health Authority whose district is included in the region or a Family Health Services Authority in relation to which it is the relevant Regional Health Authority with respect to the application of any sum paid out of those sums to the District Health Authority or the Family Health Services Authority under subsection (2) above".

Extension of functions etc. of Audit Commission to cover the health service.

1982 c. 32.

20.—(1) Part III of the Local Government Finance Act 1982 (the Audit Commission for Local Authorities in England and Wales—in this section referred to as "the Commission") shall have effect subject to the amendments in Schedule 4 to this Act, being amendments—

(a) to extend the functions of the Commission to cover health authorities and other bodies established under this Act or the principal Act;

(b) to alter the title and constitution of the Commission to reflect its wider role; and

(c) to make provision consequential on or supplemental to the amendments referred to in paragraphs (a) and (b) above.

(2) In section 98 of the principal Act (accounts and audit),—

(a) in subsection (1), in the words following paragraph (e) for the words from "appointed" to "Comptroller" there shall be substituted "appointed by the Audit Commission for Local Authorities and the National Health Service in England and Wales and the Comptroller";

(b) after subsection (2A) of that section there shall be inserted the following subsection—

"(2B) So far as relates to allotted sums paid to the members of a fund-holding practice—

(a) accounts shall be kept in such form as the Secretary of State may with the approval of the Treasury direct;

(b) the Comptroller and Auditor General may examine the accounts and the records relating to them and any report of the auditor on them;

(c) in respect of each financial year, annual accounts in such form as the Secretary of State may with the approval of the Treasury direct shall be prepared and submitted to the relevant Family Health Services Authority; and

(d) in respect of each financial year, each Family Health Services Authority shall prepare, in such form as the Secretary of State may with the approval of the Treasury

PART I

direct, and include in its own accounts, a summarised version of the accounts submitted to the Authority under paragraph (c) above.";

(c) subsection (3) (regulations of the Secretary of State with respect to audit) shall be omitted; and

(d) after subsection (4) there shall be inserted—

"(5) In subsection (2B) above "recognised fund-holding practice" and "allotted sum" have the same meaning as in section 15 of the National Health Service and Community Care Act 1990."

(3) If the person who is for the time being the auditor, within the meaning of Part III of the Local Government Finance Act 1982, in relation to the accounts of a health service body, within the meaning of that Part, has reason to believe that the body, or any officer of the body,—

1982 c. 32.

(a) is about to make, or has made, a decision which involves or would involve the incurring of expenditure which is unlawful, or

(b) is about to take, or has taken, a course of action which, if pursued to its conclusion, would be unlawful and likely to cause a loss or deficiency,

he shall refer the matter forthwith to the Secretary of State.

(4) It shall be the duty of the Commission to make, by such date as the Secretary of State may determine, an offer of employment by the Commission to each person employed in the civil service of the State in connection with the audit of the accounts of any of the bodies specified in section 98(1) of the principal Act whose name is notified to the Commission by the Secretary of State for the purposes of this subsection; and the terms of the offer must be such that they are, taken as a whole, not less favourable to the person to whom the offer is made than the terms on which he is employed on the date on which the offer is made.

(5) An offer made in pursuance of subsection (4) above shall not be revocable during the period of three months beginning with the date on which it is made.

(6) Where a person becomes an officer or servant of the Commission in consequence of subsection (4) above, then, for the purposes of the Employment Protection (Consolidation) Act 1978, his period of employment in the civil service of the State shall count as a period of employment by the Commission and the change of employment shall not break the continuity of the period of employment.

1978 c. 44.

(7) Where a person ceases to be employed as mentioned in subsection (4) above—

(a) on becoming an officer or servant of the Commission in consequence of an offer made in pursuance of that subsection, or

(b) having unreasonably refused such an offer,

he shall not, on ceasing to be so employed, be treated for the purposes of any scheme under section 1 of the Superannuation Act 1972 as having been retired on redundancy.

1972 c. 11.

(8) Without prejudice to any express amendment made by this Act, on and after the day appointed for the coming into force of this subsection, any reference in any enactment (including an enactment comprised in subordinate legislation) to the Audit Commission for Local Authorities

PART I

in England and Wales shall be construed as a reference to the Audit Commission for Local Authorities and the National Health Service in England and Wales.

Schemes for meeting losses and liabilities etc. of certain health service bodies.

21.—(1) The Secretary of State may by regulations made with the consent of the Treasury establish a scheme whereby any of the bodies specified in subsection (2) below may make provision to meet—

(a) expenses arising from any loss of or damage to their property; and

(b) liabilities to third parties for loss, damage or injury arising out of the carrying out of the functions of the bodies concerned.

(2) The bodies referred to in subsection (1) above are—

(a) health authorities;

(b) NHS trusts; and

(c) the Public Health Laboratory Service Board;

but a scheme under this section may limit the class or description of bodies which are eligible to participate in it.

(3) Without prejudice to the generality of the power conferred by subsection (1) above, a scheme under this section may—

(a) provide for the scheme to be administered by the Secretary of State or by a health authority or NHS trust specified in the scheme;

(b) require any body which participates in the scheme to make payments in accordance with the scheme; and

(c) provide for the making of payments for the purposes of the scheme by the Secretary of State.

(4) Without prejudice to any other power of direction conferred on the Secretary of State,—

(a) if the Secretary of State so directs, a body which is eligible to participate in a scheme shall do so; and

(b) where a scheme provides for it to be administered by the Secretary of State, a health authority or NHS trust shall carry out such functions in connection with the administration of the scheme by the Secretary of State as he may direct.

(5) Neither the Secretary of State nor any health authority or NHS trust administering a scheme under this section shall, by virtue of their activities under the scheme, be regarded as carrying on insurance business for the purposes of the Insurance Companies Act 1982.

1982 c. 50.

Further amendments of the principal Act

The Medical Practices Committee.

22.—(1) Section 7 of the principal Act (the Medical Practices Committee) shall be amended in accordance with this section.

(2) At the beginning of subsection (1) there shall be inserted "Subject to subsection (1A) below".

(3) After subsection (1) there shall be inserted the following subsection—

"(1A) The Secretary of State may by order make such modifications as he considers appropriate of paragraphs (a) and (b) of subsection (1) above."

(4) At the end of the section there shall be added the following subsection—

"(4) After consulting the Medical Practices Committee, the Secretary of State may give the Committee directions with respect to the exercise of its functions; and it shall be the duty of the Committee to comply with any such directions."

Distribution of general medical services.

23.—(1) In section 33 of the principal Act (distribution of general medical services) after subsection (1) there shall be inserted the following subsections—

"(1A) The Secretary of State may by order specify—

(a) the maximum number of medical practitioners with whom, in any year, all the Family Health Services Authorities for localities in England, taken as a whole, may enter into arrangements under section 29 above for the provision of general medical services; and

(b) the maximum number of medical practitioners with whom, in any year, all the Family Health Services Authorities for localities in Wales, taken as a whole, may enter into such arrangements.

(1B) An order under subsection (1A) above may contain such incidental and consequential provisions (including provisions amending this Part of this Act) as appear to the Secretary of State to be appropriate including, in particular, provisions as to the basis on which the Medical Practices Committee are to refuse applications under section 30 above in order to secure that any maximum number specified in the order is not exceeded."

(2) At the beginning of subsection (2) of that section (the Medical Practices Committee to select the persons whose applications are to be granted) there shall be inserted "Subject to subsection (2A) below" and after that subsection there shall be inserted the following subsection—

"(2A) If, in the opinion of the Medical Practices Committee, a medical practitioner is required for a particular part of the locality of a Family Health Services Authority, then, in such circumstances as may be prescribed,—

(a) the Authority (instead of the Committee) shall, in accordance with regulations, select the medical practitioner whose application they wish to be considered by the Committee; and

(b) the Committee shall not consider any application from a medical practitioner who is not so selected; and

(c) any medical practitioner who has made an application but is not so selected may appeal to the Secretary of State on a point of law;

and if the Secretary of State allows an appeal under paragraph (c) above he shall remit the application to the Authority for reconsideration."

PART I

(3) In subsection (4) of that section (applications under section 30 may be granted subject to certain conditions), after the word "but" there shall be inserted—

"(a) in granting an application shall specify, by reference to one or more prescribed conditions relating to hours or the sharing of work, the provision of general medical services for which the applicant will be entitled to be remunerated; and

(b) ";

and at the end of the subsection there shall be inserted the words "and an order under subsection (1A) above may make provision as to the extent to which account is to be taken under the order of medical practitioners whose ability to carry out remunerated work is limited by virtue of conditions imposed under paragraph (a) above".

(4) In subsection (5) of that section (appeals to the Secretary of State) for the words "such conditions" there shall be substituted "conditions under paragraph (a) or paragraph (b) of subsection (4) above" and for the words following "Secretary of State", in the first place where those words occur, there shall be substituted "on a point of law; and, if the Secretary of State allows such an appeal, he shall remit the application to the Medical Practices Committee for reconsideration".

(5) Subsection (7) of that section (directions on a successful appeal) shall be omitted.

(6) In subsection (8) of that section (matters to be taken into account) for the words from the beginning to "in any such case" there shall be substituted "In any case where medical practitioners have to be selected from a number of applicants, the Medical Practices Committee or, where subsection (2A) above applies, the Family Health Services Authority shall".

(7) In section 34 of the principal Act (regulations for Medical Practices Committee)—

(a) in paragraph (b)(ii) after the words "under section 33 above" there shall be inserted "and where such an appeal is allowed, the reconsideration of any application"; and

(b) at the end of the section there shall be added the following subsection—

"(2) Regulations under this section may make provision for, and in connection with, the variation of any condition imposed under subsection (4) or subsection (5) of section 33 above, including provision for appeals to the Secretary of State on a point of law".

(8) In the case of a medical practitioner who, on the day appointed for the coming into force of this section, is providing general medical services in accordance with arrangements under section 29 of the principal Act, regulations may make transitional provisions by virtue of which those services shall be treated for the purposes of that Act as provided subject to such of the prescribed conditions referred to in section 33(4)(a) of that Act as are determined under the regulations and, accordingly, for enabling any such condition to be varied in accordance with regulations under section 34(2) of that Act.

PART I

Limitations on right to be included on list of dental practitioners.

24.—(1) Section 36 of the principal Act (regulations as to arrangements for general dental services) shall be amended in accordance with this section.

(2) In subsection (1)(b) (regulations to include provision conferring a right, subject to certain qualifications, to be entered on a list of dental practitioners providing general dental services) for the words "subsection (2)" there shall be substituted "subsections (2) and (3)".

(3) At the end of the section there shall be added the following subsection—

"(3) Regulations may make the exercise of the right conferred by virtue of paragraph (b) of subsection (1) above subject to any provision made by or under the regulations, and, in such cases as may be prescribed, may confer a right of appeal to a prescribed body in respect of a refusal to include a dental practitioner on such a list as is referred to in paragraph (a) of that subsection."

Transfer to DHA of certain functions relating to private patients.

25.—(1) Section 65 of the principal Act (accommodation and services for private patients) shall be amended in accordance with this section.

(2) In subsection (1) (power of Secretary of State to authorise accommodation and services at hospitals to be made available for private patients etc.)—

(a) for the words from the beginning to "as he may determine", in the first place where those words occur, there shall be substituted "Subject to the provisions of this section, to such extent as they may determine, a District or Special Health Authority may make available at a hospital or hospitals for which they have responsibility accommodation and services";

(b) for any subsequent reference to the Secretary of State in the words preceding paragraph (a) there shall be substituted a reference to the District Health Authority or Special Health Authority, as the case may require; and

(c) in paragraph (a) for the words "him of any duty imposed on him by" there shall be substituted "the Authority of any function conferred on the Authority under",

(3) After subsection (1) there shall be inserted the following subsection—

"(1A) Before determining to make any accommodation or services available as mentioned in subsection (1) above, a District or Special Health Authority shall consult organisations representative of the interests of persons likely to be affected by the determination."

(4) In subsection (2)—

(a) for the words "The Secretary of State" there shall be substituted "A District or Special Health Authority"; and

(b) for the words from "to which an authorisation" to "made available" there shall be substituted "which are made available under subsection (1) above to be so made available".

(5) For subsection (3) of that section there shall be substituted the following subsection—

PART I

"(3) The Secretary of State may give directions to a District or Special Health Authority in relation to the exercise of its functions under this section; and it shall be the duty of an authority to whom directions are so given to comply with them."

Interpretation

Interpretation of Part I.
1977 c. 49.

26.—(1) Subsection (2) below has effect with respect to the interpretation of this Part of this Act and the National Health Service Act 1977 (the principal Act).

(2) In section 128 of the principal Act, in subsection (1)—

(a) after the words "this Act" there shall be inserted "and Part I of the National Health Service and Community Care Act 1990";

(b) for the definition beginning "Area Health Authority" there shall be substituted—

" "District Health Authority" means the authority for a district, whether or not its name incorporates the word "District" ";

(c) in the definition of "health service hospital" after the words "this Act" there shall be inserted "or vested in an NHS trust";

(d) after the definition of "modifications" there shall be inserted—

" "NHS contract" has the meaning assigned by section 4(1) of the National Health Service and Community Care Act 1990;

"National Health Service trust" has the meaning assigned by section 5 of the National Health Service and Community Care Act 1990 and "NHS trust" shall be construed accordingly";

(e) after the definition of "officer" there shall be inserted—

" "operational date", in relation to an NHS trust, shall be construed in accordance with paragraph 3(1)(e) of Schedule 2 to the National Health Service and Community Care Act 1990";

(f) after the definition of "patient" there shall be inserted—

" "pharmaceutical services" has the meaning assigned by section 41 of this Act";

(g) in the definition of "prescribed" after the words "this Act" there shall be inserted "or Part I of the National Health Service and Community Care Act 1990";

(h) after the definition of "prescribed" there shall be inserted—

" "primary functions" shall be construed in accordance with section 3 of the National Health Service and Community Care Act 1990"; and

(i) in the definition of "regulations" after the words "this Act" there shall be inserted "or Part I of the National Health Service and Community Care Act 1990".

(3) In this Part of this Act—

"goods" includes accommodation;

PART I

"health board" means a Health Board constituted under section 2 of the National Health Service (Scotland) Act 1978 or a Health and Social Services Board constituted under the Health and Personal Social Services (Northern Ireland) Order 1972; and

1978 c. 29.
S.I. 1972/1265 (N.I.14).

"services" includes services of any description, whether or not being services under the principal Act.

PART II

THE NATIONAL HEALTH SERVICE: SCOTLAND

Health Boards and other bodies

Health Boards, the Common Services Agency and state hospitals.

27.—(1) Subject to subsection (2) below, at the end of the day appointed for the coming into force of this subsection, any person who is a member of—

(a) a Health Board;

(b) the management committee of the Common Services Agency for the Scottish Health Service; or

(c) a State Hospital Management Committee within the meaning of the Mental Health (Scotland) Act 1984,

1984 c. 36.

shall cease to be such a member.

(2) Subsection (1) above does not apply to a person holding office as chairman of a Health Board or of a committee mentioned in subsection (1)(b) or (c) above.

(3) Schedule 1 (Health Boards) and Schedule 5 (Common Services Agency) to the National Health Service (Scotland) Act 1978 (in this Part of this Act referred to as "the 1978 Act") and Schedule 1 to the Mental Health (Scotland) Act 1984 (State Hospital Management Committees) shall be amended in accordance with Schedule 5 to this Act.

1978 c. 29.

Special Health Boards.

28. In section 2 (Health Boards) of the 1978 Act—

(a) in subsection (1)—

(i) after the words "Secretary of State" there shall be inserted the word "(a)"; and

(ii) after the words "Health Boards" there shall be inserted—

"and

(b) subject to subsections (1A) and (1C), may by order constitute boards, either for the whole of Scotland or for such parts of Scotland as he may so determine, for the purpose of exercising such of his functions under this Act as he may so determine; and those boards shall, without prejudice to subsection (1B), be called Special Health Boards.";

(b) after subsection (1) there shall be inserted the following subsections—

"(1A) An order made under subsection (1)(b) may determine an area for a Special Health Board constituted under that subsection which is the same as the areas determined—

(a) for any other Special Health Board; or

PART II

(b) for any Health Board or Health Boards constituted by an order or orders made under subsection (1)(a).

(1B) An order under subsection (1)(b) may specify the name by which a board constituted by the order shall be known.

(1C) The Secretary of State may by order provide that such of the provisions of this Act or of any other enactment, or of any orders, regulations, schemes or directions made under or by virtue of this Act or of any other enactment, as apply in relation to Health Boards shall, subject to such modifications and limitations as may be specified in the order, so apply in relation to any Special Health Board so specified."; and

(c) in subsection (2), for the word "(1)" there shall be substituted the word "(1)(a)".

Scottish advisory bodies.

29.—(1) Section 5 of the 1978 Act (Scottish Health Service Planning Council) shall cease to have effect.

(2) Section 6 of that Act (national consultative committees) shall cease to have effect.

(3) In section 7 of that Act (local health councils)—

(a) in subsection (2), the words from "by local authorities" to "and for the appointment" shall cease to have effect;

(b) in subsection (9)(d), after the words "Health Board" there shall be inserted "and from any NHS trust in their area or district"; and

(c) in subsection (9)(e), after the words "Health Board" there shall be inserted "and establishments in their area or district administered by NHS trusts".

(4) In section 8(1) of that Act (university liaison committees)—

(a) after the words "those Boards" where they first occur there shall be inserted "and any NHS trusts in the area or combined areas";

(b) for the words "the area or combined" there shall be substituted "that area or those"; and

(c) after the words "those Boards" in the second place where they occur there shall be inserted ", any such NHS trust".

(5) In section 9 of that Act (local consultative committees)—

(a) for the words from "after consultation" to "is representative" in each of subsections (1), (3) and (4) there shall be substituted "a Health Board is satisfied that a committee formed for its area is representative";

(b) for the words "Secretary of State" in the second place where they occur in subsection (1) there shall be substituted "Health Board"; and

(c) for the word "he" in each of subsections (3) and (4) there shall be substituted "the Board".

NHS contracts.

30. After section 17 of the 1978 Act there shall be inserted the following sections—

"NHS contracts.

17A.—(1) The persons or bodies mentioned in

PART II

paragraphs (a) to (e) of subsection (2) may, for the purpose of carrying out their functions under any enactment, and without prejudice to any other power they may have in that regard, enter into arrangements for the provision of goods or services to or by them with—

(a) one another; or

(b) any of the persons or bodies mentioned in paragraphs (f) to (m) of that subsection.

(2) The persons and bodies referred to in subsection (1) are—

(a) Health Boards;

(b) the Agency;

(c) the Scottish Dental Practice Board;

(d) a State Hospital Management Committee constituted under section 91 of the Mental Health (Scotland) Act 1984;

1984 c. 36.

(e) NHS trusts established under section 12A;

(f) health authorities within the meaning of section 128(1) (interpretation) of the National Health Service Act 1977;

1977 c. 49.

(g) the Dental Practice Board;

(h) the Public Health Laboratory Service Board;

(i) Family Health Services Authorities within the meaning of section 10 of the National Health Service Act 1977;

(j) recognised fund-holding practices;

(k) NHS trusts established under section 5 of the National Health Service and Community Care Act 1990;

(l) Health and Social Services Boards constituted under the Health and Personal Social Services (Northern Ireland) Order 1972; and

S.I. 1972/1265 (N.I.14).

(m) the Secretary of State.

(3) In subsection (1)—

(a) "goods" includes accommodation; and

(b) "services" includes services of any description,

and in this Act an arrangement falling within that subsection is referred to as an "NHS contract".

(4) Whether or not an arrangement which constitutes an NHS contract would, apart from this subsection, be a contract in law, it shall not be regarded for any purpose as giving rise to contractual rights or liabilities, but if any dispute arises with respect to such an arrangement, either party may refer the matter to the Secretary of State for determination under the following provisions of this section.

PART II

(5) If, in the course of negotiations intending to lead to an arrangement which will be an NHS contract, it appears to either of the prospective parties that—

(a) the terms proposed by the other party are unfair by reason that that party is seeking to take advantage of its position as the only, or the only practicable, provider of the goods or services concerned or by reason of any other unequal bargaining position as between the prospective parties to the proposed arrangement; or

(b) for any other reason arising out of the relative bargaining positions of the prospective parties any of the terms of the proposed arrangements cannot be agreed,

that party may refer the terms of the proposed arrangement to the Secretary of State for determination under the following provisions of this section.

(6) Where a reference is made to the Secretary of State under subsection (4) or (5), the Secretary of State may determine the matter himself or, if he considers it appropriate, appoint a person to consider and determine it in accordance with regulations.

(7) By his determination of a reference under subsection (5), the Secretary of State or, as the case may be, the person appointed by him under subsection (6) may specify terms to be included in the proposed arrangement and may direct that it be proceeded with; and it shall be the duty of the prospective parties to the proposed arrangement to comply with any such directions.

(8) A determination of a reference under subsection (4) may contain such directions (including directions as to payment) as the Secretary of State or, as the case may be, the person appointed under subsection (6) considers appropriate to resolve the matter in dispute; and it shall be the duty of the parties to the NHS contract in question to comply with any such directions.

(9) Without prejudice to the generality of his powers on a reference under subsection (4), the Secretary of State or, as the case may be, the person appointed by him under subsection (6) may by his determination in relation to an arrangement constituting an NHS contract vary the terms of the arrangement or bring it to an end; and where the arrangement is so varied or brought to an end—

(a) subject to paragraph (b), the variation or termination shall be treated as being effected by agreement between the parties; and

(b) directions included in the determination by virtue of subsection (8) may contain such provisions as the Secretary of State or, as the case may be, the person appointed by him under subsection (6) considers appropriate in order satisfactorily to give effect to the variation or to bring the arrangement to an end.

Reimbursement of Health Boards' costs.

17B.—(1) Where a Health Board provide goods or services under this Act for an individual for whose health care it is not their function to provide by virtue of section 2(1), in circumstances where the condition of the individual is such that he needs those goods or services and, having regard to his condition, it is not practicable, before providing them, to enter into an NHS contract for their provision, that Health Board shall be remunerated in respect of that provision by the Health Board or Health and Social Services Board which has the function, or the District or Special Health Authority which has the primary functions, of providing those goods or services to that individual.

(2) The rate of any remuneration payable by virtue of subsection (1) shall be calculated in such manner or on such basis as may be determined by the Secretary of State.

(3) In any case where—

(a) a Health Board provide goods or services for the benefit of an individual; and

(b) the provision of those goods and services is not pursuant to an NHS contract; and

(c) the individual is resident outside the United Kingdom and is of a description (being a description associating the individual with another country) specified for the purposes of this subsection by a direction made by the Secretary of State,

the Health Board shall be remunerated by the Secretary of State in respect of the provision of the goods or services at such rate or rates as he considers appropriate.

(4) In subsection (1), "Health and Social Services Board" means such a Board constituted under the Health and Personal Social Services (Northern Ireland) Order 1972."

National Health Service trusts

National Health Service trusts.

31. After section 12 of the 1978 Act there shall be inserted the following sections—

"National Health Service trusts.

12A.—(1) Subject to subsection (2), the Secretary of State may by order establish bodies, to be known as National Health Service trusts (in this Act referred to as "NHS trusts")—

(a) to assume responsibility, in accordance with this Act, for the ownership and management of hospitals or other establishments or facilities which were previously managed or provided by Health Boards or the Agency; or

PART II

(b) to provide and manage hospitals or other establishments or facilities.

(2) The Secretary of State shall by regulations provide for such consultation as may be so prescribed to be carried out by a Health Board or the Agency, before he makes an order under subsection (1).

(3) Every NHS trust—

(a) shall be a body corporate having a board of directors consisting of a chairman appointed by the Secretary of State and, subject to paragraph 5(2) of Schedule 7A, executive and non-executive directors (that is to say, directors who, subject to subsection (5), respectively are and are not employees of the trust); and

(b) shall have the functions conferred on it by an order under subsection (1) and by Schedule 7A.

(4) The functions specified in an order under subsection (1) shall include such functions as the Secretary of State considers appropriate in relation to the provision of services by the trust for one or more of the following—

(a) Health Boards; and

(b) the Agency.

(5) Regulations may make general provision with respect to—

(a) the qualifications for and the tenure of office of the chairman and directors of an NHS trust (including the circumstances in which they shall cease to hold, or may be removed from, office or may be suspended from performing the functions of the office);

(b) the persons by whom the directors and any of the officers are to be appointed and the manner of their appointment;

(c) the maximum and minimum numbers of the directors;

(d) the circumstances in which a person who is not an employee of the trust is nevertheless, on appointment as a director, to be regarded as an executive rather than as a non-executive director;

(e) the proceedings of the trust (including the validation of proceedings in the event of a vacancy or defect in appointment);

(f) the appointment, constitution and exercise of functions by committees and sub-committees of the trust (whether or not consisting of or including any members of the board); and

(g) the application of the seal of the trust and the constitution and proof of instruments.

(6) Part I of Schedule 7A shall have effect with respect to orders under subsection (1); Part II of that Schedule shall have effect, subject to subsection (7), with respect to the general duties and the powers and status of NHS trusts; the supplementary provisions of Part III of that Schedule shall have effect; and Part IV of that Schedule shall have effect with respect to the dissolution of NHS trusts.

(7) The specific powers conferred by paragraphs 14 and 15 in Part II of Schedule 7A may be exercised only to the extent that the exercise will not—

(a) interfere with the duty of the trust to comply with directions under paragraph 6 of that Schedule; and

(b) to any significant extent interfere with the performance by the trust of its obligations under any NHS contract or any obligations imposed by an order under subsection (1).

(8) The Secretary of State may by order confer on NHS trusts specific powers additional to those contained in paragraphs 10 to 15 of Schedule 7A.

Transfer of staff to NHS trusts.

12B.—(1) Subject to subsection (5), this section applies to any person who, immediately before an NHS trust's operational date—

(a) is employed by a Health Board or the Agency (in this section and section 12C referred to as a "transferor authority") to work solely at, or for the purposes of, a hospital or other establishment or facility which is to become the responsibility of the trust; or

(b) is employed by a transferor authority to work at, or for the purposes of, any such hospital, establishment or facility and is designated for the purposes of this section by a scheme made by the body specified as mentioned in paragraph 3(1)(f) of Schedule 7A.

(2) A scheme under this section shall not have effect unless approved by the Secretary of State.

(3) Subject to section 12C, the contract of employment between a person to whom this section applies and the transferor authority shall have effect from the operational date as if originally made between him and the NHS trust.

(4) Without prejudice to subsection (3)—

(a) all the transferor authority's rights, powers, duties and liabilities under or in connection with a contract to which that subsection applies shall by virtue of this section be transferred to the NHS trust on its operational date; and

(b) anything done before that date by or in relation to the transferor authority in respect of that contract or the employee shall be deemed from that date to have been done by or in relation to the NHS trust.

(5) In any case where—

(a) an order under section 12A(1) provides for the establishment of an NHS trust with effect from a date earlier than the operational date of the trust; and

(b) on or after that earlier date but before its operational date the NHS trust makes an offer of employment by the trust to a person who at that time is employed by a Health Board or the Agency to work, whether solely or otherwise, at, or for the purposes of, the hospital or other establishment or facility which is to become the responsibility of the trust; and

(c) as a result of the acceptance of the offer, the person to whom it was made becomes an employee of the NHS trust,

subsections (3) and (4) shall have effect in relation to that person's contract of employment as if he were a person to whom this section applies and any reference in those subsections to the operational date of the trust were a reference to the date on which he takes up employment with the trust.

(6) Subsections (3) and (4) are without prejudice to any right of an employee to terminate his contract of employment if a substantial change is made to his detriment in his working conditions; but no such right shall arise by reason only of the change in employer effected by this section.

(7) A scheme under this section may designate a person either individually or as a member of a class or description of employees.

Supplementary provisions as to transfer of staff.

12C.—(1) In the case of a person who falls within subsection (1)(b) of section 12B, a scheme under that section may provide that, with effect from the NHS trust's operational date, his contract of employment (in this section referred to as "his original contract") shall be treated in accordance with the scheme as divided so as to constitute—

(a) a contract of employment with the NHS trust; and

(b) a contract of employment with the transferor authority by whom he was employed before that date.

(2) Where a scheme makes provision as mentioned in subsection (1)—

(a) the scheme shall secure that the benefits to the employee under the two contracts referred to in that subsection, when taken together, are not less favourable than the benefits under his original contract;

(b) section 12B shall apply in relation to the contract referred to in subsection (1)(a) as if it were a contract transferred under that section from the transferor authority to the NHS trust;

(c) so far as necessary to preserve any rights and obligations, the contract referred to in subsection (1)(b) shall be regarded as a continuation of the employee's original contract; and

(d) for the purposes of section 146 of and Schedule 13 to the Employment Protection (Consolidation) Act 1978, the number of hours normally worked, or, as the case may be, the hours for which the employee is employed in any week under either of those contracts shall be taken to be the total of the hours normally worked or, as the case may be, for which he is employed under the two contracts taken together.

1978 c. 44.

(3) Where, as a result of the provisions of section 12B, by virtue of his employment during any period after the NHS trust's operational date—

(a) an employee has contractual rights against an NHS trust to benefits in the event of his redundancy, and

(b) he also has statutory rights against the NHS trust under Part VI of the Employment Protection (Consolidation) Act 1978 (redundancy payments),

any benefits provided to him by virtue of the contractual rights referred to in paragraph (a) shall be taken as satisfying his entitlement to benefits under Part VI of that Act.

Transfer of property rights and liabilities to NHS trusts.

12D.—(1) The Secretary of State may by order provide for the transfer to an NHS trust, with effect from such date as may be specified in the order, of such of the property, liabilities and obligations of a Health Board, the Agency or the Secretary of State as, in his opinion, need to be transferred to the NHS trust for the purpose of enabling it to carry out its functions.

PART II

(2) An order under this section may create or impose, or provide for the creation or imposition of, such new rights, liabilities or obligations in respect of what is transferred or what is retained by a Health Board or the Agency as appear to the Secretary of State to be necessary or expedient.

(3) Nothing in this section affects the power of the Secretary of State or any power of a Health Board or the Agency to transfer property, liabilities or obligations to an NHS trust otherwise than under subsection (1).

(4) Stamp duty shall not be chargeable in respect of any transfer to an NHS trust effected by virtue of an order under this section.

(5) Where an order under this section provides for the transfer—

(a) of land held on lease from a third party, that is to say, a person other than the Secretary of State; or

(b) of any other asset leased or hired from a third party or in which a third party has an interest,

the transfer shall be binding on the third party notwithstanding that, apart from this subsection, it would have required his consent or concurrence, or would have required to be intimated to him.

(6) Any property, liabilities and obligations which are to be transferred to an NHS trust shall be identified by agreement between, on the one hand, the NHS trust and, on the other hand, a Health Board or the Agency; or, in default of agreement, by direction of the Secretary of State.

(7) Where, for the purpose of a transfer pursuant to an order under this section, it becomes necessary to apportion any property, liabilities and obligations, the order may contain such provisions as appear to the Secretary of State to be appropriate for the purpose; and where any such property falls within subsection (5), the order shall contain such provisions as appear to the Secretary of State to be appropriate to safeguard the interests of third parties, including, where appropriate, provision for the payment of compensation of an amount to be determined in accordance with the order.

(8) Without prejudice to section 105(7), an order under this section may include provision for matters to be settled by arbitration by a person determined in accordance with the order.

Originating capital debt of, and other financial provisions relating to NHS trusts.

12E.—(1) Each NHS trust shall have an originating capital debt of an amount specified in an order made by the Secretary of State with the consent of the Treasury, being an amount representing, subject to subsection (2), the excess of the valuation of the assets which, on or in connection with the establishment of the trust, are or are to be transferred to it (whether before, on or after its operational date) over the amounts of the liabilities which are or are to be so transferred.

(2) In determining the originating capital debt of an NHS trust, there shall be left out of account such assets or, as the case may be, such liabilities as are, or are of a class, determined for the purposes of this section by the Secretary of State, with the consent of the Treasury.

(3) An NHS trust's originating capital debt shall be deemed to have been issued out of moneys provided by Parliament and shall constitute an asset of the Consolidated Fund.

(4) In accordance with an order under subsection (1), an NHS trust's originating capital debt shall be divided between—

(a) a loan on which interest shall be paid at such variable or fixed rates and at such times as the Treasury may determine; and

(b) public dividend capital.

(5) The loan specified in subsection (4)(a) is in this Part of this Act referred to as an NHS trust's "initial loan" and a rate of interest on the initial loan shall be determined as if section 5 of the National Loans Act 1968 had effect in respect of it and subsections (5) to (5B) of that section shall apply accordingly.

(6) Subject to subsections (4)(a) and (5), the terms of the initial loan shall be such as the Secretary of State, with the consent of the Treasury, may determine; and, in the event of the early repayment of the initial loan, the terms may require the payment of a premium or allow a discount.

(7) With the consent of the Treasury, the Secretary of State may determine the terms on which any public dividend capital forming part of an NHS trust's originating capital debt is to be treated as having been issued, and, in particular, may determine the dividend which is to be payable at any time on any public dividend capital.

(8) Schedule 7B shall have effect with respect to—

(a) borrowing by NHS trusts;

(b) the limits on their indebtedness;

(c) the payment of additional public dividend capital to them; and

(d) the application of any surplus funds of NHS trusts.

Financial obligations of NHS trusts.

12F.—(1) Every NHS trust shall ensure that its revenue is not less than sufficient, taking one financial year with another, to meet outgoings properly chargeable to revenue account.

PART II

(2) It shall be the duty of every NHS trust to achieve such financial objectives as may from time to time be set by the Secretary of State with the consent of the Treasury and as are applicable to it; and any such objectives may be made applicable to NHS trusts generally, or to a particular NHS trust or to NHS trusts of a particular description."

Further provision relating to NHS trusts.

32. After Schedule 7 to the 1978 Act there shall be inserted the Schedules set out in Schedule 6 to this Act.

Trust property of NHS trusts.

33. After section 12F of the 1978 Act (as inserted by section 31 of this Act) there shall be inserted the following section—

"Trust property of NHS trusts.

12G.—(1) Subject to subsection (2), an NHS trust shall have power to accept, hold and administer any property on trust for purposes relating to any service which it is their function to make arrangements for, administer or provide.

(2) The Secretary of State may by order make such provision as he thinks appropriate in relation to the appointment of trustees in respect of an NHS trust for the purpose of holding in trust any property which is to be so held on behalf of the trust; and any such order may include provision as to the persons by whom, the manner in which, the conditions on which and the time within which, such trustees are to be appointed.

(3) Where—

(a) section 82 applies in relation to any endowment or property which is held on trust by a Health Board; and

(b) that endowment or property is, by virtue of an order under section 12D, transferred to an NHS trust,

section 82 shall apply to the use of that endowment or property by the trust as it applied to the use thereof by the Health Board.

(4) Trustees appointed by virtue of subsection (2) shall cause proper accounts to be kept of the capital, income and expenditure vested in, received by and expended by them; and shall cause such accounts to be audited and an abstract thereof to be published in such manner as the Secretary of State may approve."

Fund-holding practices

Fund-holding practices.

34. After section 87 of the 1978 Act there shall be inserted the following sections—

"Fund-holding practices

Recognition of fund-holding practices of doctors.

87A.—(1) Any one or more medical practitioners who are providing general medical services in accordance with arrangements under section 19 may apply to the relevant Health Board for recognition as a fund-holding practice.

(2) The relevant Health Board shall not grant recognition as a fund-holding practice unless the medical practitioner or, as the case may be, each of the medical practitioners concerned fulfils such conditions as may be prescribed.

(3) Where two or more medical practitioners who wish to make an application under subsection (1) are not partners in a single partnership, section 19(8)(a) (construction of "relevant Health Board") shall apply as if the medical practitioners were practising in a single partnership.

(4) Regulations may make provision with respect to—

(a) the making of applications under subsection (1);

(b) the granting and refusal of recognition as a fund-holding practice;

(c) the conditions to be fulfilled for obtaining and continuing to be entitled to such recognition;

(d) appeals against any refusal of such recognition by a Health Board;

(e) withdrawing from, or becoming a member of, an existing recognised fund-holding practice;

(f) the continuity or otherwise of a recognised fund-holding practice in the event of the death or withdrawal of a member or the addition of a new member; and

(g) the operation of this section in a case where one or more of the medical practitioners wishing to make an application under subsection (1) is also on the medical list of a Family Health Services Authority established under section 10 of the National Health Service Act 1977,

and regulations making the provision referred to in paragraph (g) may make such modifications of the preceding provisions of this section as the Secretary of State considers appropriate.

Payments to recognised fund-holding practices.

87B.—(1) In respect of each financial year, every Health Board shall be liable to pay to the members of each recognised fund-holding practice in relation to which it is the relevant Health Board a sum determined in such manner and by reference to such factors as the Secretary of State may direct (in this section referred to as an "allotted sum").

(2) The liability to pay an allotted sum under subsection (1) may be discharged, in whole or in part, in either of the following ways—

(a) by making payments on account of the allotted sum at such times and in such manner as the Secretary of State may direct; and

PART II

(b) by discharging liabilities of the members of the practice to any other person (including, in particular, liabilities under NHS contracts);

and any reference in this section and section 87C to payment of or of a part of an allotted sum includes a reference to the discharge, in accordance with this subsection, of the whole or part of the liability to pay that sum.

(3) In any case where—

(a) a Health Board makes a payment of, or of any part of, an allotted sum to the members of a recognised fund-holding practice, and

(b) some of the individuals on the lists of patients of any of the members of the practice reside in the area of another Health Board, or in the region of a Regional Health Authority established under section 8 of the National Health Service Act 1977,

the Board making the payment shall be entitled to recover from that other Board or the Authority an amount equal to such portion of the payment as may be determined in accordance with directions given by the Secretary of State.

(4) The members of a recognised fund-holding practice may apply allotted sums only for purposes specified in regulations under subsection (5).

(5) Regulations shall make provision with respect to the purposes for which allotted sums are to be or may be applied and may make provision generally with respect to the operation of recognised fund-holding practices in relation to allotted sums; and the regulations may, in particular,—

(a) require the members of a practice to pay to the relevant Health Board out of allotted sums paid to them an amount determined in accordance with the regulations as the basic cost of the drugs, medicines and listed appliances supplied pursuant to orders given by or on behalf of members of the practice;

(b) provide that the goods and services, other than general medical services, which may be purchased by or on behalf of the members of such a practice out of allotted sums for the individuals on the lists of patients of the members of the practice shall be such as may be specified in a list approved for the purpose under the regulations; and

(c) impose a limit on the amount which may be spent out of an allotted sum on the provision of goods and services for any one individual, being a limit above which the cost of any goods and services for that individual in the financial year in question will fall to be met by the Health Board whose functions include the provision of goods and services (not necessarily the goods and services in question) to the individual concerned.

(6) In accordance with directions given by the Secretary of State, the relevant Health Board shall monitor the expenditure of the members of a recognised fund-holding practice and may institute an audit and review in any case where the Board consider it necessary to do so.

Renunciation and removal of recognition as a fund-holding practice and withholding of funds.

87C.—(1) Regulations may make provision as to the circumstances in which the members of a recognised fund-holding practice may renounce that status and such regulations may, in particular, make provision as to—

(a) the notice to be given and the number of members of the practice by whom it is to be given;

(b) the procedure to be followed; and

(c) the consequences of such a renunciation.

(2) Regulations may make provision as to the circumstances in which and the grounds on which the relevant Health Board may remove recognition from the members of a fund-holding practice,—

(a) with immediate effect; or

(b) with effect from the end of a particular financial year; or

(c) with effect from such other date as may be specified by the Health Board.

(3) Where provision is made as mentioned in subsection (2), regulations shall make provision with respect to—

(a) the procedure for removal of recognition;

(b) appeals against the removal of recognition by a Health Board; and

(c) the consequences of the removal of recognition.

(4) Without prejudice to the generality of the powers conferred by subsection (3), regulations making provision as mentioned in paragraph (c) of that subsection may—

(a) provide for the transfer of rights and obligations from the members of the fund-holding practice to one or more Health Boards determined in accordance with the regulations;

(b) provide for the recovery of sums from members of the practice; and

(c) require the members of the practice to furnish such information as may reasonably be required by the Health Board.

(5) The bringing of an appeal against the removal of recognition by a Health Board shall not be regarded as preserving the recognised status of the members of the fund-holding practice and, accordingly, subject to the outcome of the appeal, the relevant Health Board shall not be required, after the removal takes effect, to make any (or, as the case may be, any further) payment to the members of the practice of any part of the allotted sum for the financial year in question or, as the case may be, to determine and pay any allotted sum for a future financial year.

(6) Where any part of an allotted sum has been applied by the members of a recognised fund-holding practice (or any one or more of them) for purposes other than those specified in regulations under section 87B(5), regulations may make provision for and in connection with the recovery by the relevant Health Board of an amount equal to that part.

(7) Where provision is made as mentioned in subsection (6), regulations shall make provision with respect to appeals against the recovery of any amount by a Health Board."

Indicative amounts

Indicative amounts for doctors' practices.

35. After the sections inserted in the 1978 Act by section 34 above there shall be inserted the following section—

"Indicative amounts

Indicative amounts for doctors' practices.

87D.—(1) Subject to subsection (2), for each financial year every Health Board shall, by notice in writing given to each practice in relation to the members of which it is the relevant Health Board, specify an amount of money (in this Act referred to as an "indicative amount") representing the basic price of the drugs, medicines and listed appliances which, in the opinion of the Board, it is reasonable to expect will be supplied in that year pursuant to orders given by or on behalf of the members of that practice.

(2) Subsection (1) does not apply with respect to a practice which is or forms part of a fund-holding practice recognised under section 87A.

(3) For the purposes of this section, a "practice" means—

(a) a single medical practitioner who practises otherwise than in partnership; or

(b) any two or more medical practitioners who practise in partnership;

and any reference to the members of a practice shall be construed accordingly.

(4) The members of a practice shall seek to secure that, except with the consent of the relevant Health Board or for good cause, the orders for drugs, medicines and listed appliances given by them or on their behalf are such that the basic price of the items supplied pursuant to those orders in any financial year does not exceed the indicative amount notified to the practice for that year under subsection (1).

(5) For the purpose of measuring the extent to which a practice is operating within the indicative amount notified to it under subsection (1) for any financial year, a Health Board shall set against that indicative amount an amount equal to the basic price of the drugs, medicines and listed appliances supplied in that year pursuant to orders given by or on behalf of members of the practice.

(6) For the purposes of this section, regulations may make provision as to the specification of, or means of calculating, the basic price of any drugs, medicines and listed appliances.

(7) If, in the case of any practice, a member is on the medical list of a Family Health Services Authority established under section 10 of the National Health Service Act 1977 (as well as on that of a Health Board), any question whether this section applies in relation to the members of the practice shall be determined in accordance with regulations; and any such regulations may modify the preceding provisions of this section in their application to such a practice."

Audit

Accounts and audit of NHS trusts and fund-holding practices.

36.—(1) The enactments specified in Schedule 7 to this Act shall have effect subject to the amendments set out in that Schedule, being amendments—

(a) to extend the functions of the Commission for Local Authority Accounts in Scotland (in this section referred to as "the Commission") to cover Health Boards and other bodies established under the 1978 Act, the Mental Welfare Commission for Scotland and State Hospital Management Committees constituted under the Mental Health (Scotland) Act 1984;

1984 c. 36.

(b) to alter the title and constitution of the Commission to reflect its wider role; and

(c) to make provision consequential on or supplemental to the amendments referred to in paragraphs (a) and (b) above.

(2) Section 86 of the 1978 Act (keeping and audit of accounts of certain Scottish health bodies) shall be amended in accordance with the following provisions of this section.

(3) In subsection (1), for the words from the beginning to "Agency" there shall be substituted—

"(1) The following bodies, that is to say—

(a) every Health Board;

PART II

(b) the Agency; and

(c) every NHS trust,".

(4) After subsection (1) there shall be inserted the following subsections—

"(1A) So far as relates to allotted sums paid to the members of a recognised fund-holding practice—

(a) accounts shall be kept in such form as the Secretary of State may with the approval of the Treasury direct and shall be audited by auditors appointed by the Secretary of State;

(b) the Comptroller and Auditor General may examine the accounts and the records relating to them and any report of the auditor on them;

(c) in respect of each financial year, annual accounts in such form as the Secretary of State may with the approval of the Treasury direct shall be prepared and submitted to the relevant Health Board; and

(d) in respect of each financial year, each Health Board shall prepare, in such form as the Secretary of State may with the approval of the Treasury direct, and include in its own accounts, a summarised version of the accounts submitted to the Board under paragraph (c).

(1B) In preparing its annual accounts in pursuance of subsection (1), an NHS trust shall comply with any directions given by the Secretary of State with the approval of the Treasury as to—

(a) the methods and principles according to which the accounts are to be prepared; and

(b) the information to be given in the accounts."

(5) Until the day appointed for the coming into force of paragraph 14 of Schedule 7 to this Act, in subsection (2)—

(a) for the words "subsection (1)" there shall be substituted "subsections (1) and (1A)";

(b) for the words "Health Board or the Agency" there shall be substituted "body mentioned in paragraphs (a) to (c) of subsection (1) or a recognised fund-holding practice"; and

(c) for the words "Board or the Agency" there shall be substituted "body or practice".

(6) In subsection (3), for the words "Health Board and the Agency" there shall be substituted "body mentioned in paragraphs (a) to (c) of subsection (1)".

(7) In subsection (4), for the words "Health Boards and the Agency" there shall be substituted "bodies mentioned in paragraphs (a) to (c) of subsection (1)".

(8) After subsection (4) there shall be added the following subsection—

"(5) In this section "recognised fund-holding practice" and "allotted sum" have the same meaning as in section 87B."

Miscellaneous

Part II

Relationship of Health Boards and medical practitioners.

37. After subsection (7) of section 19 of the 1978 Act (arrangements and regulations for general medical services) there shall be inserted the following subsection—

"(8) In relation to a medical practitioner, any reference in this Act to the relevant Health Board shall be construed as follows—

(a) if he practises in partnership with other medical practitioners, the relevant Health Board is the Board on whose medical list the members of the practice are included and, if some are included on one Board's medical list and some on another's or if any of the members is included on the medical lists of two or more Boards, the relevant Health Board is the Board in whose area resides the largest number of individuals who are on the lists of patients of members of the practice; and

(b) in any other case, the relevant Health Board is the Board on whose medical list he is included and, if there is more than one, the Board in whose area resides the largest number of individuals who are on his list of patients."

Scottish Medical Practices Committee.

38.—(1) In section 3 of the 1978 Act (the Scottish Medical Practices Committee), after subsection (1) there shall be inserted the following subsection—

"(1A) After consulting the Medical Practices Committee, the Secretary of State may give the Committee directions with respect to the exercise of its functions; and it shall be the duty of the Committee to comply with any such directions."

(2) In Schedule 2 to the 1978 Act (constitution etc of Scottish Medical Practices Committee), after paragraph 2 there shall be inserted—

"2A. The Secretary of State may by order make such modifications as he considers appropriate of paragraphs 1 and 2."

Distribution of general medical services.

39.—(1) In section 23 of the 1978 Act (distribution of general medical services), after subsection (1) there shall be inserted the following subsections—

"(1A) The Secretary of State may by order specify the maximum number of medical practitioners with whom, in any year, all Health Boards taken as a whole may enter into arrangements under section 19 for the provision of general medical services.

(1B) An order under subsection (1A) may contain such incidental and consequential provisions (including provisions amending this Part of this Act) as appear to the Secretary of State to be appropriate including, in particular, provisions as to the basis on which the Medical Practices Committee are to refuse applications under section 20 in order to secure that any maximum number specified in the order is not exceeded."

(2) At the beginning of subsection (2) of that section (the Medical Practices Committee to select the person whose applications are to be granted) there shall be inserted "Subject to subsection (2A)" and after that subsection there shall be inserted the following subsection—

"(2A) If, in the opinion of the Medical Practices Committee, a medical practitioner is required for a particular part of the area of a Health Board, then, in such circumstances as may be prescribed,—

(a) the Board shall, in accordance with regulations, select the medical practitioner whose application they wish to be considered by the Committee; and

(b) the Committee shall not consider any application from a medical practitioner who is not so selected; and

(c) any medical practitioner who has made an application but is not so selected may appeal to the Secretary of State on a point of law;

and if the Secretary of State allows an appeal under paragraph (c) he shall remit the application to the Board for reconsideration."

(3) In subsection (4) of that section (applications under section 20 may be granted subject to certain conditions), after the word "but" there shall be inserted—

"(a) in granting an application shall specify, by reference to one or more prescribed conditions relating to hours or the sharing of work, the provision of general medical services for which the applicant will be entitled to be remunerated; and

(b)";

and at the end of the subsection there shall be inserted the words "and an order under subsection (1A) may make provision as to the extent to which account is to be taken under the order of medical practitioners whose ability to carry out remunerated work is limited by virtue of conditions imposed under paragraph (a)".

(4) In subsection (5) of that section (appeals to the Secretary of State) for the words "such conditions" there shall be substituted "conditions under paragraph (a) or (b) of subsection (4)" and for the words following "Secretary of State", in the first place where those words occur, there shall be substituted "on a point of law; and, if the Secretary of State allows such an appeal, he shall remit the application to the Medical Practices Committee for reconsideration".

(5) Subsection (7) of that section (directions on a successful appeal) shall be omitted.

(6) In subsection (8) of that section (matters to be taken into account) for the words from the beginning to "in any such case" there shall be substituted "In any case where medical practitioners have to be selected from a number of applicants, the Medical Practices Committee or, where subsection (2A) applies, the Health Board shall".

(7) In section 24 of the 1978 Act (regulations for Medical Practices Committee)—

(a) in paragraph (b)(ii) after the words "under section 23" there shall be inserted "and, where such an appeal is allowed, the reconsideration of any application"; and

(b) at the end of the section there shall be added the following subsection—

"(2) Regulations under this section may make provision for, and in connection with, the variation of any condition imposed under subsection (4) or (5) of section 23 including provision for appeals to the Secretary of State on a point of law."

(8) In the case of a medical practitioner who, on the day appointed for the coming into force of this section, is providing general medical services in accordance with arrangements under section 19 of the 1978 Act, regulations may make transitional provisions by virtue of which those services shall be treated for the purposes of that Act as provided subject to such of the prescribed conditions referred to in section 23(4)(a) of that Act as are determined under the regulations and, accordingly, for enabling any such condition to be varied in accordance with regulations under section 24(2) of that Act.

Limitations on right to be included on list of dental practitioners.

40.—(1) Section 25 of the 1978 Act (arrangements for general dental services) shall be amended in accordance with this section.

(2) In subsection (2)(b) (regulations to include provision conferring a right, subject to certain qualifications, to be entered on a list of dental practitioners providing general dental services) for the words "subsection (2A)" there shall be substituted "subsections (2A) and (2B)".

(3) After subsection (2A) there shall be inserted the following subsection—

"(2B) Regulations may make the exercise of the right conferred by virtue of paragraph (b) of subsection (2) subject to any provision made by or under the regulations, and, in such cases as may be prescribed, may confer a right of appeal to a prescribed body in respect of a refusal to include a dental practitioner on such a list as is referred to in paragraph (a) of that subsection."

Schemes for meeting losses and liabilities etc. of certain health service bodies.

41. After section 85A of the 1978 Act there shall be inserted the following section—

"Schemes for meeting losses and liabilities etc. of certain health service bodies.

85B.—(1) The Secretary of State may by regulations made with the consent of the Treasury establish a scheme whereby any of the bodies mentioned in subsection (2) may make provision to meet—

(a) expenses arising from any loss of or damage to their property; and

(b) liabilities to third parties for loss, damage (including solatium) or injury arising out of the carrying out of the functions of the bodies concerned.

(2) The bodies referred to in subsection (1) are—

(a) Health Boards;

(b) the Agency;

(c) a State Hospital Management Committee constituted under section 91 of the Mental Health (Scotland) Act 1984; and

PART II

(d) NHS trusts,

but a scheme under this section may limit the class or description of bodies which are eligible to participate in it.

(3) Without prejudice to the generality of the power conferred by subsection (1), a scheme under this section may—

(a) provide for the scheme to be administered by the Secretary of State, the Agency, or a Health Board or NHS trust specified in the scheme;

(b) require any body which participates in the scheme to make payments in accordance with the scheme; and

(c) provide for the making of payments for the purposes of the scheme by the Secretary of State.

(4) Without prejudice to any other power of direction conferred on the Secretary of State,—

(a) if the Secretary of State so directs, any body which is eligible to participate in a scheme shall do so; and

(b) where a scheme provides for it to be administered by the Secretary of State, the Agency or a Health Board or NHS trust shall carry out such functions in connection with the administration of the scheme as the Secretary of State may direct.

(5) Neither the Secretary of State nor any body administering a scheme under this section shall, by virtue of their activities under the scheme, be regarded as carrying on insurance business for the purposes of the Insurance Companies Act 1982."

PART III

COMMUNITY CARE: ENGLAND AND WALES

Provision of accommodation and welfare services

Provision of accommodation and welfare services: agency arrangements.
1948 c. 29.

42.—(1) In section 21(1) of the National Assistance Act 1948 (duties of local authorities to provide accommodation for persons aged 18 or over who are in need of care and attention by reason of age, infirmity or other circumstances)—

(a) in paragraph (a) for the word "infirmity" there shall be substituted "illness, disability"; and

(b) at the end of that paragraph there shall be added "and

(aa) residential accommodation for expectant and nursing mothers who are in need of care and attention which is not otherwise available to them".

PART III

(2) For subsections (1) and (1A) of section 26 of that Act (arrangements for provision of accommodation in premises maintained by voluntary organisations, etc.) there shall be substituted—

"(1) Subject to subsection (1A) of this section, arrangements under section 21 of this Act may include arrangements with any voluntary organisation or other person, being an organisation or person who—

(a) manages a residential care home within the meaning of Part I of the Registered Homes Act 1984, and

1984 c. 23.

(b) is registered under that Part in respect of the home or is not required to be so registered by virtue of the home being a small home or being managed or provided by an exempt body,

for the provision of accommodation in that home.

(1A) Arrangements under section 21 of this Act for the provision of residential accommodation where nursing care is provided must be arrangements made with a voluntary organisation or other person, being an organisation or person managing premises—

(a) in respect of which the organisation or other person is registered under Part II of the Registered Homes Act 1984, or

(b) which do not fall within the definition of a nursing home in section 21 of that Act by reason only of being maintained or controlled by an exempt body,

for the provision of accommodation in those premises.

(1B) Subject to subsection (1C) below no such arrangements as mentioned in subsection (1A) of this section may be made by an authority for the accommodation of any person without the consent of such District Health Authority as may be determined in accordance with regulations.

(1C) Subsection (1B) above does not apply to the making by an authority of temporary arrangements for the accommodation of any person as a matter of urgency; but, as soon as practicable after any such temporary arrangements have been made, the authority shall seek the consent required by subsection (1B) above to the making of appropriate arrangements for the accommodation of the person concerned.

(1D) No arrangements may be made by virtue of this section with a person who has been convicted of an offence under any provision of the Registered Homes Act 1984 (or any enactment replaced by that Act) or regulations made under section 16 or section 26 of that Act (or under any corresponding provisions of any such enactment)."

(3) At the end of subsection (2) of that section (under which the arrangements must provide for the local authority to make payments in respect of accommodation provided) there shall be added "and subject to subsection (3A) below the local authority shall recover from each person for whom accommodation is provided under the arrangements the amount of the refund which he is liable to make in accordance with the following provisions of this section".

PART III

(4) At the beginning of subsection (3) of that section (liability of persons for whom accommodation is provided to make refunds to the local authority) there shall be inserted "Subject to subsection (3A) below" and after that subsection there shall be inserted the following subsection—

"(3A) Where accommodation in any premises is provided for any person under arrangements made by virtue of this section and the local authority, the person concerned and the voluntary organisation or other person managing the premises (in this subsection referred to as "the provider") agree that this subsection shall apply—

(a) so long as the person concerned makes the payments for which he is liable under paragraph (b) below, he shall not be liable to make any refund under subsection (3) above and the local authority shall not be liable to make any payment under subsection (2) above in respect of the accommodation provided for him;

(b) the person concerned shall be liable to pay to the provider such sums as he would otherwise (under subsection (3) above) be liable to pay by way of refund to the local authority; and

(c) the local authority shall be liable to pay to the provider the difference between the sums paid by virtue of paragraph (b) above and the payments which, but for paragraph (a) above, the authority would be liable to pay under subsection (2) above."

(5) At the end of subsection (7) of that section (interpretation) there shall be added " "small home" means an establishment falling within section 1(4) of the Registered Homes Act 1984 and "exempt body" means an authority or body constituted by an Act of Parliament or incorporated by Royal Charter".

1984 c. 23.

(6) In section 30(1) of that Act (under which a local authority may employ certain voluntary organisations as their agents for the provision of welfare services for disabled persons) for the words from "any voluntary organisation" onwards there shall be substituted "any voluntary organisation or any person carrying on, professionally or by way of trade or business, activities which consist of or include the provision of services for any of the persons to whom section 29 above applies, being an organisation or person appearing to the authority to be capable of providing the service to which the arrangements apply".

1968 c. 46.

(7) In section 45(3) of the Health Services and Public Health Act 1968 (under which a local authority may employ certain voluntary organisations as their agents for promoting the welfare of old people) for the words from "any voluntary organisation" onwards there shall be substituted "any voluntary organisation or any person carrying on, professionally or by way of trade or business, activities which consist of or include the provision of services for old people, being an organisation or person appearing to the authority to be capable of promoting the welfare of old people".

PART III

Exclusion of powers to provide accommodation in certain cases.
1948 c. 29.

43. After section 26 of the National Assistance Act 1948 there shall be inserted—

"Exclusion of powers to provide accommodation under this Part in certain cases.

26A.—(1) Subject to subsection (3) of this section, no accommodation may be provided under section 21 or 26 of this Act for any person who immediately before the date on which this section comes into force was ordinarily resident in relevant premises.

(2) In subsection (1) "relevant premises" means—

(a) premises in respect of which any person is registered under the Registered Homes Act 1984;

(b) premises in respect of which such registration is not required by virtue of their being managed or provided by an exempt body;

(c) premises which do not fall within the definition of a nursing home in section 21 of that Act by reason only of their being maintained or controlled by an exempt body; and

(d) such other premises as the Secretary of State may by regulations prescribe;

and in this subsection "exempt body" has the same meaning as in section 26 of this Act.

(3) The Secretary of State may by regulations provide that, in such cases and subject to such conditions as may be prescribed, subsection (1) of this section shall not apply in relation to such classes of persons as may be prescribed in the regulations.

(4) The Secretary of State shall by regulations prescribe the circumstances in which persons are to be treated as being ordinarily resident in any premises for the purposes of subsection (1) of this section.

(5) This section does not affect the validity of any contract made before the date on which this section comes into force for the provision of accommodation on or after that date or anything done in pursuance of such a contract."

Charges for accommodation provided by local authorities.
1948 c. 29.

44.—(1) Section 22 of the National Assistance Act 1948 (charges for accommodation provided under Part III of that Act to be made at a standard rate fixed by the local authority subject to a minimum weekly rate prescribed under subsection (3)) shall have effect subject to the amendments specified in subsections (2) to (6) below.

(2) In subsection (1) (which relates to a person's liability to pay for accommodation) for the words from the beginning to "the accommodation" there shall be substituted "Subject to section 26 of this Act, where a person is provided with accommodation under this Part of this Act the local authority providing the accommodation shall recover from him the amount of the payment which he is liable to make".

PART III

(3) In subsection (2) (which requires the authority managing premises to fix the standard rate) after the word "payment" there shall be inserted "which a person is liable to make" and at the end of that subsection there shall be added the words "and that standard rate shall represent the full cost to the authority of providing that accommodation".

(4) In subsection (3) (which makes provision for people who are unable to pay at the standard rate)—

(a) the words "(disregarding income support)", and

(b) the words from "Provided that" to the end of the subsection,

shall be omitted.

(5) After subsection (4) (under which the Secretary of State may prescribe the minimum sum assumed to be required for a resident's personal needs in determining the rate payable by him) there shall be inserted—

"(4A) Regulations made for the purposes of subsection (4) of this section may prescribe different sums for different circumstances."

(6) In subsection (5A) (under which a local authority managing premises in which accommodation is provided for a person may limit the payments required from him for a certain period to the minimum rate prescribed under subsection (3)) for the words "the minimum weekly rate prescribed under subsection (3) above" there shall be substituted "such amount as appears to them reasonable for him to pay".

(7) In section 29 of that Act (under subsection (4)(c) of which arrangements may be made for the provision of hostels where persons for whom welfare services are provided under that section may live) after subsection (4) there shall be inserted—

"(4A) Where accommodation in a hostel is provided under paragraph (c) of subsection (4) of this section—

(a) if the hostel is managed by a local authority, section 22 of this Act shall apply as it applies where accommodation is provided under section 21;

(b) if the accommodation is provided in a hostel managed by a person other than a local authority under arrangements made with that person, subsections (2) to (4A) of section 26 of this Act shall apply as they apply where accommodation is provided under arrangements made by virtue of that section; and

(c) sections 32 and 43 of this Act shall apply as they apply where accommodation is provided under sections 21 to 26;

and in this subsection references to "accommodation" include references to board and other services, amenities and requisites provided in connection with the accommodation, except where in the opinion of the authority managing the premises or, in the case mentioned in paragraph (b) above, the authority making the arrangements their provision is unnecessary."

Recovery of charges due to local authorities for accommodation.
1983 c. 41.

45.—(1) In section 21 of the Health and Social Services and Social Security Adjudication Act 1983 (recovery of sums due to local authority where persons in residential accommodation have disposed of assets) after subsection (3) there shall be inserted—

"(3A) If the Secretary of State so directs, subsection (1) above shall not apply in such cases as may be specified in the direction."

(2) In sections 22 and 23 of that Act (which make provision as to arrears of contributions charged on interests in land in England and Wales and in Scotland respectively) after subsection (2) there shall be inserted—

"(2A) In determining whether to exercise their power under subsection (1) above and in making any determination under subsection (2) above, the local authority shall comply with any directions given to them by the Secretary of State as to the exercise of those functions."

(3) In section 24 of that Act (interest on sums charged on or secured over interests in land) for subsection (2) there shall be substituted—

"(2) The rate of interest shall be such reasonable rate as the Secretary of State may direct or, if no such direction is given, as the local authority may determine."

General provisions concerning community care services

Local authority plans for community care services.

46.—(1) Each local authority—

(a) shall, within such period after the day appointed for the coming into force of this section as the Secretary of State may direct, prepare and publish a plan for the provision of community care services in their area;

(b) shall keep the plan prepared by them under paragraph (a) above and any further plans prepared by them under this section under review; and

(c) shall, at such intervals as the Secretary of State may direct, prepare and publish modifications to the current plan, or if the case requires, a new plan.

(2) In carrying out any of their functions under paragraphs (a) to (c) of subsection (1) above, a local authority shall consult—

(a) any District Health Authority the whole or any part of whose district lies within the area of the local authority;

(b) any Family Health Services Authority the whole or any part of whose locality lies within the area of the local authority;

(c) in so far as any proposed plan, review or modifications of a plan may affect or be affected by the provision or availability of housing and the local authority is not itself a local housing authority, within the meaning of the Housing Act 1985, every such local housing authority whose area is within the area of the local authority;

1985 c. 68.

(d) such voluntary organisations as appear to the authority to represent the interests of persons who use or are likely to use any community care services within the area of the authority or the interests of private carers who, within that area, provide care to persons for whom, in the exercise of their social services functions, the local authority have a power or a duty to provide a service.

PART III

(e) such voluntary housing agencies and other bodies as appear to the local authority to provide housing or community care services in their area; and

(f) such other persons as the Secretary of State may direct.

(3) In this section—

"local authority" means the council of a county, a metropolitan district or a London borough or the Common Council of the City of London;

"community care services" means services which a local authority may provide or arrange to be provided under any of the following provisions—

1948 c. 29.

(a) Part III of the National Assistance Act 1948;

1968 c. 46.

(b) section 45 of the Health Services and Public Health Act 1968;

1977 c. 49.

(c) section 21 of and Schedule 8 to the National Health Service Act 1977; and

1983 c. 20.

(d) section 117 of the Mental Health Act 1983; and

"private carer" means a person who is not employed to provide the care in question by any body in the exercise of its functions under any enactment.

Assessment of needs for community care services.

47.—(1) Subject to subsections (5) and (6) below, where it appears to a local authority that any person for whom they may provide or arrange for the provision of community care services may be in need of any such services, the authority—

(a) shall carry out an assessment of his needs for those services; and

(b) having regard to the results of that assessment, shall then decide whether his needs call for the provision by them of any such services.

(2) If at any time during the assessment of the needs of any person under subsection (1)(a) above it appears to a local authority that he is a disabled person, the authority—

1986 c. 33.

(a) shall proceed to make such a decision as to the services he requires as is mentioned in section 4 of the Disabled Persons (Services, Consultation and Representation) Act 1986 without his requesting them to do so under that section; and

(b) shall inform him that they will be doing so and of his rights under that Act.

(3) If at any time during the assessment of the needs of any person under subsection (1)(a) above, it appears to a local authority—

(a) that there may be a need for the provision to that person by such District Health Authority as may be determined in accordance with regulations of any services under the National Health Service Act 1977, or

(b) that there may be a need for the provision to him of any services which fall within the functions of a local housing authority (within the meaning of the Housing Act 1985) which is not the local authority carrying out the assessment,

1985 c. 68.

the local authority shall notify that District Health Authority or local housing authority and invite them to assist, to such extent as is reasonable in the circumstances, in the making of the assessment; and, in making their decision as to the provision of the services needed for the person in question, the local authority shall take into account any services which are likely to be made available for him by that District Health Authority or local housing authority.

(4) The Secretary of State may give directions as to the manner in which an assessment under this section is to be carried out or the form it is to take but, subject to any such directions and to subsection (7) below, it shall be carried out in such manner and take such form as the local authority consider appropriate.

(5) Nothing in this section shall prevent a local authority from temporarily providing or arranging for the provision of community care services for any person without carrying out a prior assessment of his needs in accordance with the preceding provisions of this section if, in the opinion of the authority, the condition of that person is such that he requires those services as a matter of urgency.

(6) If, by virtue of subsection (5) above, community care services have been provided temporarily for any person as a matter of urgency, then, as soon as practicable thereafter, an assessment of his needs shall be made in accordance with the preceding provisions of this section.

(7) This section is without prejudice to section 3 of the Disabled Persons (Services, Consultation and Representation) Act 1986.

1986 c. 33.

(8) In this section—

"disabled person" has the same meaning as in that Act; and

"local authority" and "community care services" have the same meanings as in section 46 above.

Inspection of premises used for provision of community care services.

1984 c. 23.

48.—(1) Any person authorised by the Secretary of State may at any reasonable time enter and inspect any premises (other than premises in respect of which any person is registered under the Registered Homes Act 1984) in which community care services are or are proposed to be provided by a local authority, whether directly or under arrangements made with another person.

(2) Any person inspecting any premises under this section may—

(a) make such examination into the state and management of the premises and the facilities and services provided therein as he thinks fit;

(b) inspect any records (in whatever form they are held) relating to the premises, or any person for whom community care services have been or are to be provided there; and

(c) require the owner of, or any person employed in, the premises to furnish him with such information as he may request.

PART III

(3) Any person exercising the power to inspect records conferred by subsection (2)(b) above—

(a) shall be entitled at any reasonable time to have access to, and inspect and check the operation of, any computer and any associated apparatus or material which is or has been in use in connection with the records in question; and

(b) may require—

(i) the person by whom or on whose behalf the computer is or has been so used; or

(ii) any person having charge of or otherwise concerned with the operation of the computer, apparatus or material,

to give him such reasonable assistance as he may require.

(4) Any person inspecting any premises under this section—

(a) may interview any person residing there in private—

(i) for the purpose of investigating any complaint as to those premises or the community care services provided there, or

(ii) if he has reason to believe that the community care services being provided there for that person are not satisfactory; and

(b) may examine any such person in private.

(5) No person may—

(a) exercise the power conferred by subsection (2)(b) above so as to inspect medical records; or

(b) exercise the power conferred by subsection (4)(b) above,

unless he is a registered medical practitioner and, in the case of the power conferred by subsection (2)(b) above, the records relate to medical treatment given at the premises in question.

(6) Any person exercising the power of entry under subsection (1) above shall, if so required, produce some duly authenticated document showing his authority to do so.

(7) Any person who intentionally obstructs another in the exercise of that power shall be guilty of an offence and liable on summary conviction to a fine not exceeding level 3 on the standard scale.

(8) In this section "local authority" and "community care services" have the same meanings as in section 46 above.

Transfer of staff from health service to local authorities.

49.—(1) In connection with arrangements relating to community care services made by virtue of this Part of this Act, the Secretary of State may make regulations with respect to the transfer to employment by a local authority of persons previously employed by a National Health Service body.

(2) Regulations under this section may also make provision with respect to the return to employment by a National Health Service body of a person to whom the regulations previously applied on his transfer (whether from that or another National Health Service body) to employment by a local authority.

PART III

(3) Without prejudice to the generality of subsections (1) and (2) above, regulations under this section may make provision with respect to—

(a) the terms on which a person is to be employed by a local authority or National Health Service body;

(b) the period and continuity of a person's employment for the purposes of the Employment Protection (Consolidation) Act 1978;

1978 c. 44.

(c) superannuation benefits; and

(d) the circumstances in which, if a person declines an offer of employment made with a view to such a transfer or return as is referred to in subsection (1) or subsection (2) above and then ceases to be employed by a National Health Service body or local authority, he is not to be regarded as entitled to benefits in connection with redundancy.

(4) In this section—

(a) "local authority" and "community care services" have the same meaning as in section 46 above; and

(b) "National Health Service body" means a Regional, District or Special Health Authority or a National Health Service trust.

(5) Regulations under this section may make different provision with respect to different cases or descriptions of case, including different provision for different areas.

Powers of the Secretary of State as respects social services functions of local authorities.
1970 c. 42.

50. After section 7 of the Local Authority Social Services Act 1970 (local authorities to exercise social services functions under guidance of the Secretary of State) there shall be inserted the following sections—

"Directions by the Secretary of State as to exercise of social services functions.

7A.—(1) Without prejudice to section 7 of this Act, every local authority shall exercise their social services functions in accordance with such directions as may be given to them under this section by the Secretary of State.

(2) Directions under this section—

(a) shall be given in writing; and

(b) may be given to a particular authority, or to authorities of a particular class, or to authorities generally.

Complaints procedure.

7B.—(1) The Secretary of State may by order require local authorities to establish a procedure for considering any representations (including any complaints) which are made to them by a qualifying individual, or anyone acting on his behalf, in relation to the discharge of, or any failure to discharge, any of their social services functions in respect of that individual.

(2) In relation to a particular local authority, an individual is a qualifying individual for the purposes of subsection (1) above if—

(a) the authority have a power or a duty to provide, or to secure the provision of, a service for him; and

PART III

(b) his need or possible need for such a service has (by whatever means) come to the attention of the authority.

(3) A local authority shall comply with any directions given by the Secretary of State as to the procedure to be adopted in considering representations made as mentioned in subsection (1) above and as to the taking of such action as may be necessary in consequence of such representations.

(4) Local authorities shall give such publicity to any procedure established pursuant to this section as they consider appropriate.

Inquiries.

7C.—(1) The Secretary of State may cause an inquiry to be held in any case where, whether on representations made to him or otherwise, he considers it advisable to do so in connection with the exercise by any local authority of any of their social services functions (except in so far as those functions relate to persons under the age of eighteen).

1972 c. 70.

(2) Subsections (2) to (5) of section 250 of the Local Government Act 1972 (powers in relation to local inquiries) shall apply in relation to an inquiry under this section as they apply in relation to an inquiry under that section.

Default powers of Secretary of State as respects social services functions of local authorities.

1989 c. 41.

7D.—(1) If the Secretary of State is satisfied that any local authority have failed, without reasonable excuse, to comply with any of their duties which are social services functions (other than a duty imposed by or under the Children Act 1989), he may make an order declaring that authority to be in default with respect to the duty in question.

(2) An order under subsection (1) may contain such directions for the purpose of ensuring that the duty is complied with within such period as may be specified in the order as appear to the Secretary of State to be necessary.

(3) Any such direction shall, on the application of the Secretary of State, be enforceable by mandamus.

Grants to local authorities in respect of certain social services.

7E. The Secretary of State may, with the approval of the Treasury, make grants out of money provided by Parliament towards any expenses of local authorities incurred—

(a) in connection with the exercise of their social services functions in relation to persons suffering from mental illness; or

(b) in making payments, in accordance with directions given by the Secretary of State to voluntary organisations which provide care and services for persons who are, have been, or are likely to become dependent upon alcohol or drugs.

PART IV

COMMUNITY CARE: SCOTLAND

Power of Secretary of State to give directions.
1968 c. 49.

51. After subsection (1) of section 5 (powers of Secretary of State) of the Social Work (Scotland) Act 1968 (in this Part of this Act referred to as "the 1968 Act") there shall be inserted the following subsection—

PART IV

"(1A) Without prejudice to subsection (1) above, the Secretary of State may issue directions to local authorities, either individually or collectively, as to the manner in which they are to exercise any of their functions under this Act or any of the enactments mentioned in section 2(2) of this Act; and a local authority shall comply with any direction made under this subsection."

Local authority plans for, and complaints in relation to, community care services in Scotland.

52. After section 5 of the 1968 Act there shall be inserted the following sections—

"Local authority plans for community care services.

5A.—(1) Within such period after the day appointed for the coming into force of this section as the Secretary of State may direct, and in accordance with the provisions of this section, each local authority shall prepare and publish a plan for the provision of community care services in their area.

(2) Each local authority shall from time to time review any plan prepared by them under subsection (1) above, and shall, in the light of any such review, prepare and publish—

(a) any modifications to the plan under review; or

(b) if the case requires, a new plan.

(3) In preparing any plan or carrying out any review under subsection (1) or, as the case may be, subsection (2) above the authority shall consult—

(a) any Health Board providing services under the National Health Service (Scotland) Act 1978 in the area of the authority;

1978 c. 29.

(b) in so far as the plan or, as the case may be, the review may affect or be affected by the provision or availability of housing, every district council in the area of the authority;

(c) such voluntary organisations as appear to the authority to represent the interests of persons who use or are likely to use any community care services within the area of the authority or the interests of private carers who, within that area, provide care to persons for whom, in the exercise of their functions under this Act or any of the enactments mentioned in section 2(2) of this Act, the local authority have a power or a duty to provide, or to secure the provision of, a service;

(d) such voluntary housing agencies and other bodies as appear to the authority to provide housing or community care services in their area; and

(e) such other persons as the Secretary of State may direct.

PART IV

(4) In this section—

"community care services" means services, other than services for children, which a local authority are under a duty or have a power to provide, or to secure the provision of, under Part II of this Act or section 7 (functions of local authorities), 8 (provision of after-care services) or 11 (training and occupation of the mentally handicapped) of the Mental Health (Scotland) Act 1984; and

"private carer" means a person who is not employed to provide the care in question by any body in the exercise of its functions under any enactment.

Complaints procedure.

5B.—(1) Subject to the provisions of this section, the Secretary of State may by order require local authorities to establish a procedure whereby a person, or anyone acting on his behalf, may make representations (including complaints) in relation to the authority's discharge of, or failure to discharge, any of their functions under this Act, or any of the enactments referred to in section 2(2) of this Act, in respect of that person.

(2) For the purposes of subsection (1) of this section, "person" means any person for whom the local authority have a power or a duty to provide, or to secure the provision of, a service, and whose need or possible need for such a service has (by whatever means) come to the attention of the authority.

(3) An order under subsection (1) of this section may be commenced at different times in respect of such different classes of person as may be specified in the order.

(4) In relation to a child, representations may be made by virtue of subsection (1) above by the child, or on his behalf by—

(a) his parent;

(b) any person having parental rights in respect of him;

(c) any local authority foster parent; or

(d) any other person appearing to the authority to have a sufficient interest in the child's wellbeing to warrant his making representations on the child's behalf.

(5) In this section—

"child" means a child under the age of 18 years; and

"parent" and "parental rights" have the same meaning as in section 8 (interpretation) of the Law Reform (Parent and Child) (Scotland) Act 1986.

PART IV

(6) A local authority shall comply with any directions given by the Secretary of State as to the procedure to be adopted in considering representations made as mentioned in subsection (1) of this section and as to the taking of such action as may be necessary in consequence of such representations.

(7) Every local authority shall give such publicity to the procedure established under this section as they consider appropriate."

Inspection of premises providing accommodation.

53.—(1) Section 6 of the 1968 Act (supervision of establishments and places providing accommodation etc) shall be amended as follows.

(2) In subsection (1) after "place" insert "the facilities and services provided therein".

(3) In subsection (1), for the words "required to be kept therein" there shall be substituted "(in whatever form they are held) relating to the place or to any person for whom services have been or are provided there".

(4) After subsection (2) there shall be inserted the following subsections—

"(2A) Any such person may require the owner of, or any person employed in, the establishment or place in question to furnish him with such information as he may request.

(2B) In exercising the power to inspect records and registers under this section a person—

(a) shall be entitled at any reasonable time to have access to, and inspect and check the operation of, any computer and any associated apparatus or material which is or has been in use in connection with the records or register in question; and

(b) may require—

(i) the person by whom or on whose behalf the computer is or has been so used; or

(ii) any person having charge of or otherwise concerned with the operation of the computer, apparatus or material,

to give him such reasonable assistance as he may require.

(2C) In exercising the power to inspect places under this section a person—

(a) may interview any person residing there in private—

(i) for the purpose of investigating any complaint as to that place or the services provided there; or

(ii) if he has reason to believe that the services being provided there for that person are not satisfactory; and

(b) may examine any such person in private.

(2D) No person may—

(a) exercise the power to inspect records or registers under subsection (1) or (2) above so as to inspect medical records; or

PART IV

(b) exercise the power conferred by subsection (2C)(b) above,

unless he is a registered medical practitioner and, in the case of the power conferred by subsection (1) or (2) above, the records or register relate to medical treatment given at the place in question."

Inquiries.

54. After section 6 of the 1968 Act there shall be inserted the following section—

"Inquiries.

6A.—(1) The Secretary of State may cause an inquiry to be held into the functions of a local authority under this Act or any of the enactments mentioned in section 2(2) of this Act, except in so far as those functions relate to persons under the age of 18.

(2) The Secretary of State may, before an inquiry is commenced, direct that it shall be held in private, but where no such direction has been given the person holding the inquiry may if he thinks fit hold it or any part of it in private.

1973 c. 65.

(3) Subsections (2) to (8) of section 210 of the Local Government (Scotland) Act 1973 (powers in relation to local inquiries) shall apply in relation to an inquiry under this section as they apply in relation to a local inquiry under that section."

Duty of local authority to make assessment of needs.

55. After section 12 of the 1968 Act there shall be inserted the following section—

"Duty of local authority to assess needs.

12A.—(1) Subject to the provisions of this section, where it appears to a local authority that any person for whom they are under a duty or have a power to provide, or to secure the provision of, community care services may be in need of any such services, the authority—

(a) shall make an assessment of the needs of that person for those services; and

(b) having regard to the results of that assessment, shall then decide whether the needs of that person call for the provision of any such services.

(2) Before deciding, under subsection (1)(b) of this section, that the needs of any person call for the provision of nursing care, a local authority shall consult a medical practitioner.

(3) If, while they are carrying out their duty under subsection (1) of this section, it appears to a local authority that there may be a need for the provision to any

person to whom that subsection applies—

(a) of any services under the National Health Service (Scotland) Act 1978 by the Health Board—

(i) in whose area he is ordinarily resident: or

(ii) in whose area the services to be supplied by the local authority are, or are likely, to be provided: or

PART IV

(b) of any services which fall within the functions of a housing authority (within the meaning of section 130 (housing) of the Local Government (Scotland) Act 1973) which is not the local authority carrying out the assessment,

the local authority shall so notify that Health Board or housing authority, and shall request information from them as to what services are likely to be made available to that person by that Health Board or housing authority; and, thereafter, in carrying out their said duty, the local authority shall take into account any information received by them in response to that request.

(4) Where a local authority are making an assessment under this section and it appears to them that the person concerned is a disabled person, they shall—

(a) proceed to make such a decision as to the services he requires as is mentioned in section 4 of the Disabled Persons (Services, Consultation and Representation) Act 1986 without his requesting them to do so under that section; and

1986 c. 33.

(b) inform him that they will be doing so and of his rights under that Act.

(5) Nothing in this section shall prevent a local authority from providing or arranging for the provision of community care services for any person without carrying out a prior assessment of his needs in accordance with the preceding provisions of this section if, in the opinion of the authority, the condition of that person is such that he requires those services as a matter of urgency.

(6) If, by virtue of subsection (5) of this section, community care services have been provided for any person as a matter of urgency, then, as soon as practicable thereafter, an assessment of his needs shall be made in accordance with the preceding provisions of this section.

(7) This section is without prejudice to section 3 of the said Act of 1986.

(8) In this section—

"community care services" has the same meaning as in section 5A of this Act;

"disabled person" has the same meaning as in the said Act of 1986; and "medical practitioner" means a fully registered person within the meaning of section 55 (interpretation) of the Medical Act 1983."

Residential accommodation with nursing and provision of care and after-care.

56. After section 13 of the 1968 Act there shall be inserted the following sections—

PART IV

"Residential accommodation with nursing

Residential accommodation with nursing.

13A.—(1) Without prejudice to section 12 of this Act, a local authority shall make such arrangements as they consider appropriate and adequate for the provision of suitable residential accommodation where nursing is provided for persons who appear to them to be in need of such accommodation by reason of infirmity, age, illness or mental disorder, dependency on drugs or alcohol or being substantially handicapped by any deformity or disability.

(2) The arrangements made by virtue of subsection (1) above shall be made with a voluntary or other organisation or other person, being an organisation or person managing premises which are—

1938 c. 73.

(a) a nursing home within the meaning of section 10(2)(a) of the Nursing Homes Registration (Scotland) Act 1938 in respect of which that organisation or person is registered or exempt from registration under that Act; or

1984 c. 36.

(b) a private hospital registered under section 12 of the Mental Health (Scotland) Act 1984,

for the provision of accommodation in those premises.

(3) The provisions of section 6 of this Act apply in relation to premises where accommodation is provided for the purposes of this section as they apply in relation to establishments provided for the purposes of this Act.

Provision of care and after-care

Provision of care and after-care.

13B.—(1) Subject to subsection (2) below, a local authority may, with the approval of the Secretary of State, and shall, if and to the extent that the Secretary of State so directs, make arrangements for the purpose of the prevention of illness, the care of persons suffering from illness, and the after-care of such persons.

(2) The arrangements which may be made under subsection (1) above do not include arrangements in respect of medical, dental or nursing care, or health visiting."

Exclusion of powers to provide accommodation in certain cases.

57. After section 86 of the 1968 Act there shall be inserted the following section—

"Exclusion of powers to provide accommodation in certain cases.

86A.—(1) Subject to subsection (3) below, no accommodation may be provided under this Act for any person who, immediately before the date on which this section comes into force, was ordinarily resident in relevant premises.

(2) In subsection (1) above "relevant premises" means—

(a) any establishment in respect of which a person is registered under section 62 of this Act;

(b) any nursing home within the meaning of the Nursing Homes Registration (Scotland) Act 1938 in respect of which a person is registered or exempt from registration under that Act;

PART IV 1938 c. 73.

(c) any private hospital registered under section 12 of the Mental Health (Scotland) Act 1984; and

1984 c. 36.

(d) such other premises as the Secretary of State may by regulations prescribe.

(3) The Secretary of State may by regulations provide that in such cases and subject to such conditions as may be prescribed subsection (1) above shall not apply in relation to such classes of persons as may be prescribed in the regulations.

(4) The Secretary of State shall by regulations prescribe the circumstances in which persons are to be treated as being ordinarily resident in any premises for the purposes of subsection (1) above.

(5) This section does not affect the validity of any contract made before the date on which this section comes into force for the provision of accommodation on or after that date or anything done in pursuance of such a contract."

Power of Secretary of State to make grants.

58. After section 92 of the 1968 Act there shall be inserted the following section—

"Power of the Secretary of State to make grants.

92A. The Secretary of State may, with the approval of the Treasury, make grants out of money provided by Parliament towards any expenses of local authorities in respect of their functions under—

(a) Part II of this Act; and

(b) sections 7 and 8 of the Mental Health (Scotland) Act 1984,

1984 c. 36.

in relation to persons suffering from mental illness."

Parliamentary disqualification.
1975 c. 24.

PART V

MISCELLANEOUS AND GENERAL

59.—(1) In Schedule 1 to the House of Commons Disqualification Act 1975 (offices disqualifying for membership of the House of Commons), in Part III for the entry which begins "Chairman in receipt of remuneration of any Regional Health Authority" there shall be substituted the following entry—

"Chairman or any member, not being also an employee, of any Regional Health Authority, District Health Authority, Family Health Services Authority or special health authority which is a relevant authority for the purposes of paragraph 9(1) of Schedule 5 to the National Health Service Act 1977."

(2) In the said Part III there shall be inserted (at the appropriate place) the following entry—

"Chairman or non-executive member of a National Health Service trust established under the National Health Service and Community Care Act 1990 or the National Health Service (Scotland) Act 1978".

(3) In the said Part III—

(a) in the entry which begins "Paid Chairman of a Health Board", for the words "Paid Chairman" there shall be substituted "Chairman or any member, not being also an employee,";

(b) in the entry which begins "Chairman of the Management Committee of the Common Services Agency" after the word "Chairman" there shall be inserted "or any member, not being also an employee,"; and

1984 c. 36.

(c) in the entry relating to the Chairman of a committee constituted under section 91 of the Mental Health (Scotland) Act 1984, after the word "Chairman" there shall be inserted "or any member, not being also an employee".

Removal of Crown immunities.

60.—(1) Subject to the following provisions of this section, on and after the day appointed for the coming into force of this subsection, no health service body shall be regarded as the servant or agent of the Crown or as enjoying any status, immunity or privilege of the Crown; and so far as concerns land in which the Secretary of State has an interest, at any time when—

1977 c. 49.
1988 c. 49.
1978 c. 29.

(a) by virtue of directions under any provision of the National Health Service Act 1977, the Mental Health (Scotland) Act 1984 or the Health and Medicines Act 1988 or by virtue of orders under section 2 or section 10 of the National Health Service (Scotland) Act 1978, powers of disposal or management with respect to the land are conferred on a health service body, or

(b) the land is otherwise held, used or occupied by a health service body,

the interest of the Secretary of State shall be treated for the purposes of any enactment or rule of law relating to Crown land or interests as if it were an interest held otherwise than by the Secretary of State (or any other emanation of the Crown).

(2) In Schedule 8 to this Act—

(a) Part I has effect to continue certain exemptions for health service bodies and property held, used or occupied by such bodies;

(b) the amendments in Part II have effect, being amendments consequential on subsection (1) above; and

(c) the transitional provisions in Part III have effect in connection with the operation of subsection (1) above.

(3) Where, as a result of the provisions of subsection (1) above, by virtue of his employment during any period after the day appointed for the coming into force of that subsection—

(a) an employee has contractual rights against a health service body to benefits in the event of his redundancy, and

(b) he also has statutory rights against the health service body under Part VI of the Employment Protection (Consolidation) Act 1978 (redundancy payments),

PART V

1978 c. 44.

any benefits provided to him by virtue of the contractual rights referred to in paragraph (a) above shall be taken as satisfying his entitlement to benefits under the said Part VI.

(4) Nothing in subsection (1) above affects the extent of the expression "the services of the Crown" where it appears in—

(a) Schedule 1 to the Registered Designs Act 1949 (provisions as to the use of registered designs for the services of the Crown etc.); and

1949 c. 88.

(b) sections 55 to 59 of the Patents Act 1977 (use of patented inventions for the services of the Crown);

1977 c. 37.

and, accordingly, services provided in pursuance of any power or duty of the Secretary of State under Part I of the National Health Service Act 1977 or Part I or Part III of the National Health Service (Scotland) Act 1978 shall continue to be regarded as included in that expression, whether the services are in fact provided by a health service body, a National Health Service trust or any other person.

1977 c. 49.
1978 c. 29.

(5) The Secretary of State may by order made by statutory instrument provide that, in relation to any enactment contained in a local Act and specified in the order, the operation of subsection (1) above shall be excluded or modified to the extent specified in the order.

(6) No order shall be made under subsection (5) above unless a draft of it has been laid before, and approved by a resolution of, each House of Parliament.

(7) In this section "health service body" means—

(a) a health authority, within the meaning of the National Health Service Act 1977;

(b) a Health Board or Special Health Board constituted under section 2 of the National Health Service (Scotland) Act 1978;

(c) a State Hospital Management Committee constituted under section 91 of the Mental Health (Scotland) Act 1984;

1984 c. 36.

(d) a Family Health Services Authority;

(e) the Common Services Agency for the Scottish Health Service;

(f) the Dental Practice Board;

(g) the Scottish Dental Practice Board; and

(h) the Public Health Laboratory Service Board.

Health service bodies: taxation. 1988 c. 1.

61.—(1) In Part XII of the Income and Corporation Taxes Act 1988 (special classes of companies and business: miscellaneous businesses and bodies) after section 519 there shall be inserted the following section—

"Health service bodies.

519A.—(1) A health service body—

(a) shall be exempt from income tax in respect of its income, and

PART V

(b) shall be exempt from corporation tax,

and, so far as the exemption from income tax conferred by this subsection calls for repayment of tax, effect shall be given thereto by means of a claim.

(2) In this section "health service body" means—

(a) a health authority, within the meaning of the National Health Service Act 1977;

(b) a National Health Service trust established under Part I of the National Health Service and Community Care Act 1990;

(c) a Family Health Services Authority;

(d) a Health Board or Special Health Board, the Common Services Agency for the Scottish Health Service and a National Health Service trust respectively constituted under sections 2, 10 and 12A of the National Health Service (Scotland) Act 1978;

(e) a State Hospital Management Committee constituted under section 91 of the Mental Health (Scotland) Act 1984;

(f) the Dental Practice Board;

(g) the Scottish Dental Practice Board; and

(h) the Public Health Laboratory Service Board."

1979 c. 14.

(2) In section 149B of the Capital Gains Tax Act 1979 (miscellaneous exemptions from tax) in subsection (3) after the words "section 519 of the Taxes Act 1988" there shall be inserted "and a health service body, within the meaning of section 519A of that Act".

1978 c. 29.

1891 c. 39.

(3) Where any conveyance, transfer or lease is made or agreed to be made to a National Health Service trust established under Part I of the National Health Service and Community Care Act 1990 or the National Health Service (Scotland) Act 1978, no stamp duty shall be chargeable by virtue of any of the following headings in Schedule 1 to the Stamp Act 1891—

(a) "Conveyance or Transfer on Sale",

(b) "Conveyance or Transfer of any kind not hereinbefore described",

(c) "Lease or Tack",

on the instrument by which the conveyance, transfer or lease, or the agreement for it, is effected.

(4) At the end of section 27 of the Value Added Tax Act 1983 (application to Crown) there shall be added the following subsection—

1983 c. 55.

"(5) For the purposes of subsection (4) above a National Health Service trust established under Part I of the National Health Service and Community Care Act 1990 or the National Health Service (Scotland) Act 1978 shall be regarded as a body of persons exercising functions on behalf of a Minister of the Crown."

(5) At the end of Schedule 3 to the Inheritance Tax Act 1984 (gifts for national purposes) there shall be added—

"A health service body, within the meaning of section 519A of the Income and Corporation Taxes Act 1988".

PART V

1984 c. 51.

Clinical Standards Advisory Group.

62.—(1) There shall be established in accordance with this section a Clinical Standards Advisory Group (in this section referred to as "the Advisory Group") which shall have the following functions—

(a) in accordance with a request made by the Health Ministers or any one of them, to provide advice on the standards of clinical care for, and the access to and availability of services to, national health service patients and, in this connection, to carry out such investigations into such matters (if any) and to make such reports in relation thereto as the Health Ministers may require;

(b) in accordance with a request made by one or more health service bodies, to provide advice on, to carry out investigations into and to report on the standards of clinical care for, and the access to and availability of services to, national health service patients for whom services are or are to be provided by or on behalf of the body or bodies concerned; and

(c) such other functions as may be prescribed by regulations.

(2) The Advisory Group shall consist of a chairman and other members appointed by the Health Ministers and regulations may—

(a) require that one or more members of the Advisory Group shall be appointed from persons nominated by such body or bodies as may be specified in the regulations; and

(b) provide that one or more of the members who are not appointed from persons so nominated must fulfil such conditions or hold such posts as may be so specified.

(3) Regulations may make provision as to—

(a) the appointment, tenure and vacation of office of the chairman and members of the Advisory Group;

(b) the appointment of and the exercise of functions by committees and sub-committees of the Advisory Group (including committees and sub-committees consisting wholly or partly of persons who are not members of the Advisory Group);

(c) the procedure of the Advisory Group and any committees or sub-committees thereof; and

(d) the attendance at meetings of the Advisory Group or any committee or sub-committee thereof of persons appointed by the Health Ministers and the extent of their participation in such meetings.

(4) Proceedings of the Advisory Group, or of any committee or sub-committee of the Advisory Group, shall not be invalidated by any vacancy in membership or by any defect in a member's appointment or qualifications.

(5) The Health Ministers—

(a) may pay to the chairman and members of the Advisory Group, or of any committee or sub-committee of the Advisory Group or any persons appointed as mentioned in subsection (3)(d) above, such sums by way of remuneration and travelling and other allowances as the Health Ministers, with the consent of the Treasury, may determine;

PART V

(b) shall make available to the Advisory Group and to any committee or sub-committee thereof such staff and other services or facilities as are necessary to enable them to carry out their functions; and

(c) shall defray such expenditure as is reasonably incurred by the Advisory Group in carrying out their functions.

(6) Where the Advisory Group carry out an investigation or make a report in accordance with a request made by a health service body, that body shall reimburse, in such manner as the Health Ministers may determine, so much of the expenditure incurred by them under paragraphs (a) and (c) of subsection (5) above as they certify as being attributable to the carrying out of that investigation or the making of that report.

(7) In this section—

"clinical care" means any action which is taken in connection with the diagnosis of illness or the care or treatment of a patient, and which is taken solely in consequence of the exercise of clinical judgment;

"the Health Ministers" means the Secretaries of State respectively concerned with health in England, in Wales and in Scotland;

"health service body" means—

1977 c. 49.

(i) a health authority, within the meaning of the National Health Service Act 1977,

1978 c. 29.

(ii) a Health Board or Special Health Board constituted under section 2 of the National Health Service (Scotland) Act 1978,

1984 c. 36.

(iii) a State Hospital Management Committee constituted under section 91 of the Mental Health (Scotland) Act 1984.

(iv) the Common Services Agency for the Scottish Health Service,

(v) a National Health Service trust constituted under Part I of this Act or under the National Health Service (Scotland) Act 1978, and

(vi) a Family Health Services Authority;

"national health service patient" means any person for whom any services are or are to be provided by or on behalf of a health service body;

"regulations" means regulations made by the Health Ministers and any such regulations may make different provision for different cases or descriptions of case, including different provision for different areas; and

"services" means services provided—

(a) in England and Wales, by virtue of directions under section 13 or section 14 of the National Health Service Act 1977 or section 5 of this Act; or

(b) in Scotland, by a health service body under Part I or Part III of the National Health Service (Scotland) Act 1978; or

(c) pursuant to an NHS contract, as defined in section 4(1) of this Act or section 17A of the National Health Service (Scotland) Act 1978.

PART V

1978 c. 29.

Repeal of remaining provisions of Health Services Act 1976.

1976 c. 83.

63.—(1) Part III (control of hospital building outside National Health Service) and Part IV (supplementary and general) of the Health Services Act 1976 shall cease to have effect.

(2) Notwithstanding the repeal of Part III of the Health Services Act 1976 by this Act,—

(a) that Part shall continue to have effect in relation to any authorisation granted by the Secretary of State under section 13(2) of that Act which is in force when that repeal takes effect; and

(b) the amendment made by section 19(4)(b) of that Act shall continue to have effect.

Financial provisions.

64.—(1) There shall be paid out of moneys provided by Parliament—

(a) any sums required by the Secretary of State for making loans to a National Health Service trust;

(b) any sums required by the Secretary of State for fulfilling a guarantee of a sum borrowed by a National Health Service trust;

(c) any amount paid as public dividend capital under paragraph 5 of Schedule 3 to this Act;

(d) any expenses of the Secretary of State under this Act; and

(e) any increase attributable to this Act in the sums so payable under any other enactment.

(2) Any sums received by the Secretary of State under this Act shall be paid into the Consolidated Fund.

Regulations, orders and directions.

65.—(1) Any power to make regulations conferred by this Act shall be exercisable by statutory instrument, and any such statutory instrument shall be subject to annulment in pursuance of a resolution of either House of Parliament.

1977 c. 49.

(2) In section 126 of the National Health Service Act 1977 (orders and regulations and directions) in each of subsections (2) to (4) after the words

"this Act" there shall be inserted "or Part I of the National Health Service and Community Care Act 1990" and at the end of that section there shall be added the following subsection—

"(5) Without prejudice to the generality of subsection (4) above, any power which may be exercised as mentioned in paragraphs (a) and (b) of that subsection may make different provision for different areas."

Amendments and repeals.

66.—(1) Schedule 9 to this Act, which contains minor amendments and amendments consequential on the provisions of this Act, shall have effect.

(2) The enactments specified in Schedule 10 to this Act, which include some that are spent, are hereby repealed to the extent specified in the third column of that Schedule.

PART V

Short title, commencement and extent.

67.—(1) This Act may be cited as the National Health Service and Community Care Act 1990.

(2) This Act, other than this section, shall come into force on such day as the Secretary of State may by order made by statutory instrument appoint, and different days may be so appointed for different provisions or for different purposes and for different areas or descriptions of areas.

(3) An order under subsection (2) above may contain such transitional provisions and savings (whether or not involving the modification of any statutory provision) as appear to the Secretary of State necessary or expedient in connection with the provisions brought into force.

(4) Part I of this Act, other than section 15(4), does not extend to Scotland; Part II, other than section 34, and Part IV of this Act do not extend to England and Wales; and Part III of this Act, other than subsections (3) and (4) of section 42, subsections (1) and (3) to (6) of section 44 and section 45, does not extend to Scotland.

(5) This Act, other than sections 59 and 61, does not extend to Northern Ireland.

(6) The Secretary of State may by order made by statutory instrument provide that so much of this Act as extends to England and Wales shall apply to the Isles of Scilly with such modifications, if any, as are specified in the order and, except as provided in pursuance of this subsection, Parts I and III of this Act do not apply to the Isles of Scilly.

SCHEDULES

SCHEDULE 1

Sections 1 and 2.

HEALTH AUTHORITIES AND FAMILY HEALTH SERVICES AUTHORITIES

PART I

MEMBERSHIP OF REGIONAL AND DISTRICT HEALTH AUTHORITIES

Regional health authorities

1.—(1) A Regional Health Authority shall consist of—

(a) a chairman appointed by the Secretary of State;

(b) a prescribed number of members appointed by him;

(c) the chief officer of the authority;

(d) such other officers as may be prescribed; and

(e) not more than a prescribed number of other officers of the authority appointed by the chairman and the members specified in paragraphs (b) and (c) above.

(2) Except in so far as regulations otherwise provide, no person who is an officer of the authority may be appointed under sub-paragraph (1)(b) above; and, without prejudice to any provision made by virtue of paragraph 12(a) of Schedule 5 to the principal Act (regulations as to appointment and tenure)—

(a) at least one of the persons appointed under sub-paragraph (1)(b) above must hold a post in a university with a medical or dental school; and

(b) regulations may provide that all or any of the other persons appointed under sub-paragraph (1)(b) above must fulfil prescribed conditions or hold posts of a prescribed description.

District health authorities

2.—(1) A District Health Authority for a district in England shall consist of—

(a) a chairman appointed by the Secretary of State;

(b) a prescribed number of members appointed by the Regional Health Authority whose region includes the district in question;

(c) the chief officer of the authority;

(d) such other officers as may be prescribed; and

(e) not more than a prescribed number of other officers of the authority appointed by the chairman and the members specified in paragraphs (b) and (c) above.

(2) Except in so far as regulations otherwise provide, no person who is an officer of the authority may be appointed under sub-paragraph (1)(b) above; and, without prejudice to any provision made by virtue of paragraph 12(a) of Schedule 5 to the principal Act (regulations as to appointment and tenure), but subject to sub-paragraph (3) below, regulations may provide that all or any of the persons appointed under sub-paragraph (1)(b) above must fulfil prescribed conditions or hold posts of a prescribed description.

(3) In the case of a prescribed authority, at least one of the persons appointed under sub-paragraph (1)(b) above must hold a post in a university with a medical or dental school.

3.—(1) A District Health Authority for a district in Wales shall consist of—

(a) a chairman appointed by the Secretary of State;

(b) a prescribed number of members appointed by him;

SCH. 1

(c) the chief officer of the authority;

(d) such other officers as may be prescribed; and

(e) not more than a prescribed number of other officers of the authority appointed by the chairman and the members specified in paragraphs (b) and (c) above.

(2) Sub-paragraphs (2) and (3) of paragraph 2 above apply in relation to sub-paragraph (1) above as they apply in relation to sub-paragraph (1) of that paragraph.

PART II

MEMBERSHIP OF FAMILY HEALTH SERVICES AUTHORITIES

4.—(1) A Family Health Services Authority in England shall consist of—

(a) a chairman appointed by the Secretary of State;

(b) a prescribed number of members appointed by the Regional Health Authority which (in accordance with Section 15(1A) of the principal Act) is the relevant Regional Health Authority in relation to the Family Health Services Authority; and

(c) the chief officer of the Authority;

(d) such other officers as may be prescribed;

and, if the Secretary of State so directs, the Authority shall also include not more than a prescribed number of other officers of the Authority appointed by the chairman and the members appointed under paragraphs (b) and (c) above.

(2) No person who is an officer of the Authority may be appointed under sub-paragraph (1)(b) above; and, without prejudice to any provision made by virtue of paragraph 12(a) of Schedule 5 to the principal Act (regulations as to appointment and tenure), regulations may provide that all or any of the persons appointed under sub-paragraph (1)(b) above must fulfil prescribed conditions or hold posts of a prescribed description.

5.—(1) A Family Health Services Authority in Wales shall consist of—

(a) a chairman appointed by the Secretary of State;

(b) a prescribed number of members appointed by him; and

(c) the chief officer of the Authority;

(d) such other officers as may be prescribed;

and, if the Secretary of State so directs, the Authority shall also include not more than a prescribed number of other officers of the Authority appointed by the chairman and the members appointed under paragraphs (b) and (c) above.

(2) Sub-paragraph (2) of paragraph 4 above applies in relation to sub-paragraph (1) above as it applies in relation to sub-paragraph (1) of that paragraph.

PART III

AMENDMENTS OF PART III OF SCHEDULE 5 TO THE PRINCIPAL ACT

6. In paragraph 8 of Schedule 5, (corporate status) the words "Area Health Authority" shall be omitted.

7.—(1) In paragraph 9 of that Schedule (pay and allowances), in sub-paragraph (1) after the words "chairman of an authority" there shall be inserted "and to any member of a relevant authority who is appointed by the Secretary of State or a Regional Health Authority".

SCH. 1

(2) At the end of the paragraph there shall be added the following sub-paragraph—

"(7) In sub-paragraph (1) above "relevant authority" means—

(a) a Regional Health Authority, a District Health Authority or a Family Health Services Authority; or

(b) any special health authority which is specified in Schedule 1 to the Authorities for London Post-Graduate Teaching Hospitals (Establishment and Constitution) Order 1982, in the Board of Governors of the Eastman Dental Hospital (Establishment and Constitution) Order 1984 or in any other provision of an order under this Act which specifies an authority for the purposes of this sub-paragraph."

S.I.1982/314.

S.I.1984/188

8. In paragraph 10 of that Schedule (staff) at the end of sub-paragraph (1A) there shall be added the words "and a direction under that sub-paragraph may relate to a particular officer or class of officer specified in the direction".

9. In paragraph 12 of that Schedule (regulations as to tenure of office, committees and sub-committees and procedure etc. of authorities)—

(a) at the end of paragraph (a) there shall be added the words "and any members of a committee or sub-committee of an authority who are not members of the authority";

(b) after paragraph (a) there shall be inserted the following paragraph—

"(aa) the circumstances in which a member of an authority who is (or is to be regarded as) an officer of the authority may be suspended from performing his functions as a member"; and

(c) in paragraph (b) after the word "appointment" there shall be inserted "and constitution".

10. After paragraph 12 of that Schedule there shall be inserted the following paragraph—

"12A. Regulations made by virtue of this Schedule or Schedule 1 to the National Health Service and Community Care Act 1990 may make provision (including provision modifying those Schedules) to deal with cases where the post of chief officer or any other officer of an authority is held jointly by two or more persons or where the functions of such an officer are in any other way performed by more than one person."

SCHEDULE 2

Section 5.

NATIONAL HEALTH SERVICE TRUSTS

PART I

ORDERS UNDER SECTION 5(1)

1.—(1) Any reference in this Part of this Schedule to an order is a reference to an order under section 5(1) of this Act establishing an NHS trust or any subsequent order under that provision amending or revoking a previous order.

(2) An order shall be made by statutory instrument.

2. The provisions made by an order shall be in conformity with any general provision made by regulations under section 5(7) of this Act.

3.—(1) Without prejudice to any amendment made by a subsequent order, the first order to be made in relation to any NHS trust shall specify—

(a) the name of the trust;

SCH. 2

(b) the functions of the trust;

(c) the number of executive directors and non-executive directors;

(d) where the trust is to be regarded as having a significant teaching commitment, a provision to secure the inclusion in the non-executive directors referred to in paragraph (c) above of a person appointed from a university with a medical or dental school specified in the order;

(e) the operational date of the trust, that is to say, the date on which the trust is to begin to undertake the whole of the functions conferred on it; and

(f) if a scheme is to be made under section 6 of this Act, the health authority which is to make the scheme.

(2) For the purposes of sub-paragraph (1)(d) above, an NHS trust is to be regarded as having a significant teaching commitment in the following cases—

(a) if the trust is established to assume responsibility for the ownership and management of a hospital or other establishment or facility which, in the opinion of the Secretary of State, has a significant teaching and research commitment; and

(b) in any other case, if the Secretary of State so provides in the order.

(3) In a case where the order contains a provision made by virtue of sub-paragraph (1)(d) above and a person who is being considered for appointment by virtue of that provision—

(a) is employed by the university in question, and

(b) would also, apart from this sub-paragraph, be regarded as employed by the trust,

his employment by the trust shall be disregarded in determining whether, if appointed, he will be a non-executive director of the trust.

(4) An order shall specify the accounting date of the trust.

4.—(1) An order may require a Regional, District or Special Health Authority to make staff, premises and other facilities available to an NHS trust pending the transfer or appointment of staff to or by the trust and the transfer of premises or other facilities to the trust.

(2) An order making provision under this paragraph may make provision with respect to the time when the Regional, District or Special Health Authority's functions under the provision are to come to an end.

5.—(1) An order may provide for the establishment of an NHS trust with effect from a date earlier than the operational date of the trust and, during the period between that earlier date and the operational date, the trust shall have such limited functions for the purpose of enabling it to begin to operate satisfactorily with effect from the operational date as may be specified in the order.

(2) If an order makes the provision referred to in sub-paragraph (1) above, then, at any time during the period referred to in that sub-paragraph, the NHS trust shall be regarded as properly constituted (and may carry out its limited functions accordingly) notwithstanding that, at that time, all or any of the executive directors have not yet been appointed.

(3) If an order makes the provision referred to in sub-paragraph (1) above, the order may require a Regional, District or Special Health Authority to discharge such liabilities of the NHS trust as—

(a) may be incurred during the period referred to in that sub-paragraph; and

(b) are of a description specified in the order.

PART II

DUTIES, POWERS AND STATUS

Specific duties

6.—(1) An NHS trust shall carry out effectively, efficiently and economically the functions for the time being conferred on it by an order under section 5(1) of this Act and by the provisions of this Schedule and, with respect to the exercise of the powers conferred by section 5(10) of this Act and paragraphs 10 to 15 below, shall comply with any directions given to it by the Secretary of State, whether of a general or a particular nature.

(2) An NHS trust shall comply with any directions given to it by the Secretary of State with respect to all or any of the following matters—

(a) the qualifications of persons who may be employed as officers of the trust;

(b) the employment, for the purpose of performing functions specified in the direction, of officers having qualifications or experience of a description so specified;

(c) the manner in which officers of the trust are to be appointed;

(d) prohibiting or restricting the disposal of, or of any interest in, any asset which, at the time the direction is given, the Secretary of State reasonably considers to have a value in excess of such sum as may be specified in an order under section 5(1) of this Act and in respect of which the Secretary of State considers that the interests of the National Health Service require that the asset should not be disposed of;

(e) compliance with guidance or directions given (by circular or otherwise) to health authorities, or particular descriptions of health authorities; and

(f) the implementation of awards relating to the distinction or merit of medical practitioners or dental practitioners or any class or classes of such practitioners.

7.—(1) For each accounting year an NHS trust shall prepare and send to the Secretary of State an annual report in such form as may be determined by the Secretary of State.

(2) At such time or times as may be prescribed, an NHS trust shall hold a public meeting at which its audited accounts and annual report and any report on the accounts made pursuant to subsection (3) of section 15 of the Local Government Finance Act 1982 shall be presented.

1982 c. 32.

(3) In such circumstances and at such time or times as may be prescribed, an NHS trust shall hold a public meeting at which such document as may be prescribed shall be presented.

8. An NHS trust shall furnish to the Secretary of State such reports, returns and other information, including information as to its forward planning, as, and in such form as, he may require.

9.—(1) An NHS trust shall be liable to pay—

(a) to the chairman and any non-executive director of the trust remuneration of an amount determined by the Secretary of State, not exceeding such amount as may be approved by the Treasury;

(b) to the chairman and any non-executive director of the trust such travelling and other allowances as may be determined by the Secretary of State with the approval of the Treasury;

SCH. 2

(c) to any member of a committee or sub-committee of the trust who is not also a director such travelling and other allowances as may be so determined.

(2) If an NHS trust so determines in the case of a person who is or has been a chairman of the trust, the trust shall be liable to pay such pension, allowances or gratuities to or in respect of him as may be determined by the Secretary of State with the approval of the Treasury.

(3) Different determinations may be made under sub-paragraph (1) or sub-paragraph (2) above in relation to different cases or descriptions of cases.

Specific powers

10. In addition to carrying out its other functions, an NHS trust may, as the provider, enter into NHS contracts.

11. An NHS trust may undertake and commission research and make available staff and provide facilities for research by other persons.

12. An NHS trust may—

(a) provide training for persons employed or likely to be employed by the trust or otherwise in the provision of services under the principal Act; and

(b) make facilities and staff available in connection with training by a university or any other body providing training in connection with the health service.

13. An NHS trust may enter into arrangements for the carrying out, on such terms as seem to the trust to be appropriate, of any of its functions jointly with any Regional, District or Special Health Authority, with another NHS trust or with any other body or individual.

14. According to the nature of its functions, an NHS trust may make accommodation or services or both available for patients who give undertakings (or for whom undertakings are given) to pay, in respect of the accommodation or services (or both) such charges as the trust may determine.

15. For the purpose of making additional income available in order better to perform its functions, an NHS trust shall have the powers specified in section 7(2) of the Health and Medicines Act 1988 (extension of powers of Secretary of State for financing the Health Service).

1988 c. 49.

General powers

16.—(1) Subject to Schedule 3 to this Act, an NHS trust shall have power to do anything which appears to it to be necessary or expedient for the purpose of or in connection with the discharge of its functions, including in particular power—

(a) to acquire and dispose of land and other property;

(b) to enter into such contracts as seem to the trust to be appropriate;

(c) to accept gifts of money, land or other property, including money, land or other property to be held on trust, either for the general or any specific purposes of the NHS trust or for all or any purposes relating to the health service; and

(d) to employ staff on such terms as the trust thinks fit.

(2) The reference in sub-paragraph (1)(c) above to specific purposes of the NHS trust includes a reference to the purposes of a specific hospital or other establishment or facility which is owned and managed by the trust.

17.—(1) Without prejudice to the generality of paragraph 16 above, for or in respect of such of its employees as it may determine, an NHS trust may make such arrangements for providing pensions, allowances or gratuities as it may determine; and such arrangements may include the establishment and administration, by the trust or otherwise, of one or more pension schemes.

(2) The reference in sub-paragraph (1) above to pensions, allowances or gratuities to or in respect of employees of an NHS trust includes a reference to pensions, allowances or gratuities by way of compensation to or in respect of any of the trust's employees who suffer loss of office or employment or loss or diminution of emoluments.

Status

18. An NHS trust shall not be regarded as the servant or agent of the Crown or, except as provided by this Act, as enjoying any status, immunity or privilege of the Crown; and an NHS trust's property shall not be regarded as property of, or property held on behalf of, the Crown.

PART III

SUPPLEMENTARY PROVISIONS

Re-imbursement for health services work carried out otherwise than under NHS contract

19.—(1) In any case where an NHS trust provides goods or services for the benefit of an individual and—

(a) the provision of those goods or services is not pursuant to an NHS contract, and

(b) the condition of the individual is such that he needs those goods or services and, having regard to his condition, it is not practicable before providing them to enter into an NHS contract for their provision, and

(c) the provision of those goods or services is within the primary functions of a District Health Authority or is a function of a health board,

the trust shall be remunerated by that Authority or health board in respect of the provision of the goods or services in question.

(2) The rate of any remuneration payable by virtue of sub-paragraph (1) above shall be calculated in such manner or on such basis as may be determined by the Secretary of State.

20. In any case where an NHS trust provides goods or services for the benefit of an individual and—

(a) the provision of those goods or services is not pursuant to an NHS contract, and

(b) the individual is resident outside the United Kingdom and is of a description (being a description associating the individual with another country) specified for the purposes of this paragraph by a direction made by the Secretary of State,

the trust shall be remunerated by the Secretary of State in respect of the provision of the goods or services in question at such rate or rates as he considers appropriate.

Supply of goods and services by local authorities

21. In section 28 of the principal Act (supply of goods and services by local authorities) in subsection (3) after the words "health authorities", in each place where they occur, there shall be inserted "and NHS trusts", and at the end there shall be added "and the National Health Service and Community Care Act 1990".

SCH. 2

Making of charges

22. In each of sections 81 (charges for more expensive supplies) and 82 (charges for repairs and replacement necessitated by an act or omission of the person supplied etc.) of the principal Act, in paragraph (a)—

(a) after the words "Secretary of State" there shall be inserted "or an NHS trust"; and

(b) after the word "him" there shall be inserted "or, as the case may be, by the trust".

Power to raise money by appeals etc.

23.—(1) In section 96A of the principal Act (power of health authorities etc. to raise money etc. by appeals, collections etc.) in subsection (1), after the word "authority", in each place where it occurs, there shall be inserted "or NHS trust".

(2) In subsections (3), (4) and (7) to (9) of that section, for the words "authority or Board", in each place where they occur, there shall be substituted "authority, NHS trust or Board".

(3) In subsection (5), of that section, for the words from "Area or District" onwards there shall be substituted "body responsible for the hospital if that body and the special trustees agree; and in this subsection the body responsible for a hospital is,—

(a) in the case of a hospital vested in a NHS trust, that trust; and

(b) in any other case, the District Health Authority exercising functions on behalf of the Secretary of State in respect of the hospital".

(4) After subsection (5) of that section there shall be inserted the following subsection—

"(5A) Where property is given in pursuance of this section on trust for any purposes of an NHS trust for which trustees have been appointed under section 11(1) of the National Health Service and Community Care Act 1990, then, if those trustees and the NHS trust agree, the property may be held, administered and applied by those trustees instead of by the NHS trust."

(5) In subsection (6) of that section for the words "or to special trustees" there shall be substituted "to an NHS trust or to special trustees or trustees for an NHS trust".

Accounts and audit

24.—(1) In section 98 of the principal Act (accounts and audit), in subsection (1) after paragraph (bb) there shall be inserted—

"(bbb) every NHS trust".

(2) After subsection (2A) of that section there shall be inserted—

"(2B) in preparing its annual accounts in pursuance of subsection (2) above, an NHS trust shall comply with any directions given by the Secretary of State with the approval of the Treasury as to—

(a) the methods and principles according to which the accounts are to be prepared; and

(b) the information to be given in the accounts."

Protection of members and officers

25. In section 125 of the principal Act (protection of members and officers of health authorities etc.)—

(a) for paragraph (b) there shall be substituted—

SCH. 2

"(b) an NHS trust"; and

(b) at the end there shall be added "and the National Health Service and Community Care Act 1990".

Compulsory acquisition

26.—(1) An NHS trust may be authorised to purchase land compulsorily for the purposes of its functions by means of an order made by the trust and confirmed by the Secretary of State.

(2) Subject to sub-paragraph (3) below, the Acquisition of Land Act 1981 shall apply to the compulsory purchase of land under this paragraph.

1981 c. 67.

(3) No order shall be made by an NHS trust under Part II of the Acquisition of Land Act 1981 with respect to any land unless the proposal to acquire the land compulsorily—

(a) has been submitted to the Secretary of State in such form and together with such information as he may require; and

(b) has been approved by him.

Use and development of consecrated land and burial grounds

27. Section 128 of the Town and Country Planning Act 1971 (use and development of consecrated land and burial grounds) applies to consecrated land and land comprised in a burial ground, within the meaning of that section, which an NHS trust holds for any of its purposes as if—

1971 c. 78.

(a) that land had been acquired by the trust as mentioned in subsection (1) of that section; and

(b) the trust were a statutory undertaker, within the meaning of that Act.

Instruments etc.

28.—(1) The fixing of the seal of an NHS trust shall be authenticated by the signature of the chairman or of some other person authorised either generally or specially by the trust for that purpose and of one other director.

(2) Any document purporting to be a document duly executed under the seal of an NHS trust shall be received in evidence and shall, unless the contrary is proved, be deemed to be so executed.

(3) A document purporting to be signed on behalf of an NHS trust shall be received in evidence and shall, unless the contrary is proved, be deemed to be so signed.

PART IV
DISSOLUTION

29.—(1) The Secretary of State may by order made by statutory instrument dissolve an NHS trust.

(2) An order under this paragraph may be made—

(a) on the application of the NHS trust concerned; or

(b) if the Secretary of State considers it appropriate in the interests of the health service.

(3) Except where it appears to the Secretary of State necessary to make an order under this paragraph as a matter of urgency, no such order shall be made until after the completion of such consultation as may be prescribed.

SCH. 2

30.—(1) If an NHS trust is dissolved under this Part of this Schedule, the Secretary of State may by order transfer or provide for the transfer to—

(a) the Secretary of State, or

(b) a health authority, or

(c) another NHS trust,

of such of the property, rights and liabilities of the NHS trust which is dissolved as in his opinion is appropriate; and any such order may include provisions corresponding to those of section 8 of this Act.

(2) An order under this paragraph may make provision in connection with the transfer of staff employed by or for the purposes of the NHS trust which is dissolved; and such an order may include provisions corresponding to those of sections 6 and 7 of this Act, including provision for the making of a scheme by such health authority or other body as may be specified in the order.

(3) No order shall be made under this paragraph until after completion of such consultation as may be prescribed.

31. Without prejudice to the generality of paragraph 30 above, if an NHS trust is dissolved under this Part of this Schedule, the Secretary of State or such other NHS trust or health authority as he may direct shall undertake the responsibility for the continued payment of any such pension, allowances or gratuities as, by virtue of paragraph 9(2) or paragraph 17 above, would otherwise have been the responsibility of the trust which has been dissolved.

32. An NHS trust may not be dissolved or wound up except in accordance with this Part of this Schedule.

Section 9.

SCHEDULE 3

FINANCIAL PROVISIONS RELATING TO NHS TRUSTS

Borrowing

1.—(1) Subject to the provisions of this paragraph and to any limit imposed under the following provisions of this Schedule, for the purpose of its functions an NHS trust may borrow (both temporarily, by way of overdraft, and longer term) from the Secretary of State or from any other person.

(2) An NHS trust may not mortgage or charge any of its assets or in any other way use any of its assets as security for a loan.

(3) Except with the consent of the Secretary of State, an NHS trust may not borrow in any currency other than sterling; and the Secretary of State shall not give his consent to any such borrowing except with the approval of the Treasury.

(4) Interest on any sums borrowed from the Secretary of State by an NHS trust shall be paid at such variable or fixed rates and at such times as the Treasury may determine.

1968 c. 13.

(5) A rate of interest under sub-paragraph (4) above shall be determined as if section 5 of the National Loans Act 1968 had effect in respect of it and subsections (5) to (5B) of that section shall apply accordingly.

(6) Subject to sub-paragraphs (4) and (5) above, the terms on which any sums are borrowed from the Secretary of State by an NHS trust shall be such as he may determine; and, in the event of the early repayment of any sums so borrowed, such terms may require the payment of a premium or allow a discount.

Guarantees of borrowing

2.—(1) The Secretary of State may guarantee, in such manner and on such conditions as, with the approval of the Treasury, he considers appropriate, the repayments of the principal of and the payment of interest on any sums which an NHS trust borrows from a person other than the Secretary of State.

(2) Immediately after a guarantee is given under this paragraph, the Secretary of State shall lay a statement of the guarantee before each House of Parliament.

(3) Where any sum is issued for fulfilling a guarantee so given, the Secretary of State shall lay before each House of Parliament a statement relating to that sum as soon as possible after the end of each financial year beginning with that in which the sum is issued and ending with that in which all liability in respect of the principal of the sum and in respect of interest on it is finally discharged.

(4) If any sums are issued in fulfilment of a guarantee given under this paragraph, the NHS trust concerned shall make to the Secretary of State, at such times and in such manner as the Secretary of State may from time to time direct,—

(a) payments of such amounts as the Secretary of State with the consent of the Treasury so directs in or towards repayment of the sums so issued; and

(b) payments of interest, at such rates as the Secretary of State with the consent of the Treasury so directs, on what is outstanding for the time being in respect of sums so issued.

Limits on indebtedness

3.—(1) The aggregate of all sums borrowed by NHS trusts established to assume responsibility for the ownership and management of, or to provide and manage, hospitals or other establishments or facilities which are situated in England shall not exceed £5,000 million or such other sum not exceeding £10,000 million as may be specified by order made by the Secretary of State with the consent of the Treasury.

(2) The aggregate of all sums borrowed by NHS trusts established to assume responsibility for the ownership and management of, or to provide and manage, hospitals or other establishments or facilities which are situated in Wales shall not exceed £300 million or such other sum not exceeding £600 million as may be specified by order made by the Secretary of State with the consent of the Treasury.

(3) The references in sub-paragraphs (1) and (2) above to sums borrowed do not include a reference to NHS trusts' initial loans.

4. Any power to make an order under paragraph 3 above shall be exercisable by statutory instrument which shall be subject to annulment in pursuance of a resolution of the House of Commons.

Additional public dividend capital

5.—(1) If the Secretary of State, with the consent of the Treasury, considers it appropriate to do so, he may, instead of making a loan to an NHS trust under paragraph 1 above, pay an amount to the trust as public dividend capital.

(2) Section 9 of this Act shall apply to public dividend capital paid to an NHS trust under this paragraph as it applies to public dividend capital forming part of the trust's originating capital debt.

SCH. 3

Surplus funds

6. If it appears to the Secretary of State that any amount standing in the reserves of an NHS trust is surplus to its foreseeable requirements, the trust shall, if the Secretary of State with the approval of the Treasury and after consultation with the trust so directs, pay that amount into the Consolidated Fund.

Investment

7. An NHS trust may not invest any money held by it except in securities of the Government of the United Kingdom or in such other manner as the Secretary of State may with the consent of the Treasury approve.

Section 20.

SCHEDULE 4

AMENDMENTS OF PART III OF THE LOCAL GOVERNMENT FINANCE ACT 1982

1.—(1) In section 11 (establishment of Audit Commission), in subsection (1) after the words "Local Authorities" there shall be inserted "and the National Health Service".

(2) In subsection (2) of that section,—

(a) for the word "thirteen" there shall be substituted "fifteen";

(b) for the word "seventeen" there shall be substituted "twenty"; and

(c) for paragraphs (a) and (b) there shall be substituted the words "such organisations and other bodies as appear to him to be appropriate".

2.—(1) In section 12 (accounts subject to audit), in subsection (2) after paragraph (e) there shall be inserted—

"(ea) a body specified in section 98(1) of the National Health Service Act 1977".

(2) After subsection (3) of that section there shall be inserted the following subsections—

"(3A) This section also applies to the accounts of the members of a recognised fund-holding practice so far as they relate to allotted sums paid to them, and subject to subsection (3B) and section 16(1A) below, any reference in this Part of this Act to the accounts of a body shall be construed, in relation to the members of a fund-holding practice, as a reference to such of their accounts as relate to allotted sums so paid.

(3B) In such circumstances and to such extent as regulations made by the Secretary of State so provide, this Part of this Act shall not apply to the accounts for any year of the members of a recognised fund-holding practice if those accounts are submitted to a Family Health Services Authority and summarised in that Authority's accounts.

(3C) In subsection (3A) above "allotted sums" has the same meaning as in section 15 of the National Health Service and Community Care Act 1990."

(3) After subsection (4) of that section there shall be inserted the following subsection—

"(5) Any reference in this Part of this Act to a health service body is a reference to a body specified in section 98(1) of the National Health Service Act 1977 or to the members of a recognised fund-holding practice as mentioned in subsection (3A) above."

3.—(1) In section 13 (appointment of auditors), in each of subsections (3) and (4), after the word "body", in the first place where it occurs, there shall be inserted "other than a health service body".

SCH. 4

(2) In subsection (5) of that section after the words "Secretary of State" there shall be inserted "or is a person for the time being approved by the Secretary of State, acting on the recommendation of the Commission".

(3) After subsection (5) of that section there shall be inserted the following subsection—

"(5A) The Secretary of State shall not approve any person for the purposes of subsection (5) above after 31st March 1996 but, subject to the withdrawal of his approval after that date, any person who is so approved immediately before that date shall continue to be so approved after that date."

4.—(1) In section 14 (code of audit practice), at the end of subsection (1) there shall be added "and a different code may be prepared with respect to the audit of the accounts of health service bodies as compared with the code applicable to the accounts of other bodies".

(2) At the end of the section there shall be added the following subsection—

"(7) In the application of subsection (6) above to a code which relates to the accounts of health services bodies,—

(a) if the code relates only to those accounts, the reference to associations of local authorities shall be construed as a reference to organisations connected with the health service, within the meaning of the National Health Service Act 1977; and

(b) if the code relates also to the accounts of other bodies, that reference shall be construed as including a reference to such organisations."

5. In section 15 (general duties of auditors), in subsection (1)(a) after the words "section 23 below" there shall be inserted "or, in the case of a health service body, directions under subsection (2) or subsection (2B) of section 98 of the National Health Service Act 1977".

6. In section 16 (auditor's rights to obtain documents and information) after subsection (1) there shall be inserted the following subsection—

"(1A) In the case of a recognised fund-holding practice the reference in subsection (1) above to documents includes a reference to documents relating to all the accounts and records of the members of the practice, whether or not relating to the allotted sum, within the meaning of that section."

7. In section 17 (public inspection of accounts and right of challenge), in subsection (1) after the words "Part of this Act" there shall be inserted "other than the audit of the accounts of a health service body".

8. In section 18 (auditor's reports), in subsection (4) after the word "Commission" there shall be inserted "and, in the case of a health service body, to the Secretary of State".

9. In section 19 (declaration that item of account is unlawful), in subsection (1) after the words "Part of this Act" there shall be inserted "other than the audit of the accounts of a health service body".

10. In section 20 (recovery of amount not accounted for etc.), in subsection (1) after the words "Part of this Act" there shall be inserted "other than the audit of the accounts of a health service body".

SCH. 4

11. In section 21 (fees for audit), after subsection (2) there shall be inserted the following subsection—

"(2A) In the application of subsection (2) above to the audit of the accounts of a health service body, the reference to associations of local authorities shall be construed as a reference to organisations connected with the health service."

12.—(1) In section 22 (extraordinary audit), at the beginning of each of subsections (1) and (3) there shall be inserted "Subject to subsection (4A) below".

(2) After subsection (4) of that section there shall be inserted the following subsection—

"(4A) Subsection (1)(a) above does not apply in relation to the accounts of a health service body; and in the application of subsection (3) above to an extraordinary audit of any such accounts for the words "15 to 20 above, except subsections (1) and (2) of section 17" there shall be substituted "15, 16, and 18 above"."

13. In section 23 (regulations as to accounts), in subsection (1) after the words "this Part of this Act" there shall be inserted "other than health service bodies".

14. In section 24 (right of local government elector to inspect accounts etc.), in subsection (1) after the words "Part of this Act" there shall be inserted "other than a health service body".

15. At the end of section 25 (audit of accounts of officers) there shall be inserted the following subsection —

"(2) In the application of subsection (1) above to an officer of a health service body for the words "15 to 24" there shall be substituted "15, 16, 18, 21 and 22"."

16. In section 25A (power of auditor to issue prohibition order), in subsection (1) after the words "Part of this Act", in the first place where they occur, there shall be inserted "other than a health service body".

17. In section 25D (power of auditor to apply for judicial review), in subsection (1) after the word "body", in the first place where it occurs, there shall be inserted "other than a health service body".

18.—(1) In section 26 (studies for improving economy etc. in services), at the end of subsection (3) there shall be added "and, in the case of studies relating to a health service body, shall, on request, furnish to the Comptroller and Auditor General, all material relevant to the studies".

(2) At the end of subsection (4) of that section there shall be added "and, in the case of any health service bodies, the Commission shall also consult the Secretary of State and the Comptroller and Auditor General".

19.—(1) In section 27 (reports on impact of statutory provisions etc.), in subsection (1) after the words "Part of this Act" there shall be inserted "other than health service bodies".

(2) At the end of that section there shall be added the following subsection—

"(6) Notwithstanding that the services provided by health service bodies are excluded from the scope of studies under this section, in undertaking or promoting studies under section 26(1) above relating to a health service body, the Commission may take into account the implementation by the body of—

(a) any particular statutory provision or provisions, and

(b) any directions or guidance given by the Secretary of State (whether pursuant to any such provision or otherwise),

but the power conferred by this subsection shall not be construed as entitling the Commission to question the merits of the policy objectives of the Secretary of State."

20.—(1) In section 29 (miscellaneous functions of Commission), at the end of subsection (2) there shall be added "or, in the case of a health service body, such other organisations as appear to the body to be appropriate".

(2) At the end of subsection (3) of that section there shall be added "or the National Health Service".

21. In section 30 (restriction on disclosure of information), in subsection (1)(b) after the words "Part of this Act" there shall be inserted "or, in the case of a health service body, for the purposes of the functions of the Secretary of State and the Comptroller and Auditor General under the National Health Service Act 1977".

22.—(1) In section 33 (commencement and transitional provisions) after subsection (4) there shall be inserted the following subsection—

"(4A) The Secretary of State may by regulations provide for any statutory provision not contained in this Part of this Act to continue to apply on and after the day appointed for the coming into force of paragraph 22 of Schedule 4 to the National Health Service and Community Care Act 1990 in relation to accounts for any period beginning before that day of health service bodies, with such modifications, additions and omissions as may be prescribed by the regulations; and different provision may be made by such regulations in relation to the accounts of bodies of different descriptions and in relation to the accounts for different periods.

(2) In subsection (5) of that section (provision of working capital to the Commission) for the words "second appointed day", in the second place where they occur, there shall be substituted "day appointed for the coming into force of paragraph 22 of Schedule 4 to the National Health Service and Community Care Act 1990" and at the end of the subsection there shall be added the words "with respect to its functions in relation to health service bodies".

23. In section 36 (interpretation), in subsection (1),—

(a) in the definition of "the Commission" after the words "Local Authorities" there shall be inserted "and the National Health Service"; and

(b) after that definition there shall be inserted—

"health service body" has the meaning assigned by section 12(5) above;

"recognised fund-holding practice" shall be construed in accordance with section 14 of the National Health Service and Community Care Act 1990".

24.—(1) In Schedule 3 (provisions as to the Commission), in paragraph 3(3) for the word "and", in the last place where it occurs, there shall be substituted "or, as the case may require, such organisations connected with the health service as appear to him to be appropriate and (in either case)".

(2) At the beginning of paragraph 9 there shall be inserted "Subject to sub-paragraph (2) below" and at the end of the paragraph there shall be inserted—

SCH. 4

"(2) Sub-paragraph (1) above shall apply separately with respect to the functions of the Commission in relation to health service bodies and its functions in relation to other bodies."

Section 27.

SCHEDULE 5

HEALTH BOARDS, THE COMMON SERVICES AGENCY AND STATE HOSPITALS

Health Boards

1. Schedule 1 to the 1978 Act shall be amended in accordance with paragraphs 2 to 7 below.

2. After paragraph 2 of that Schedule (membership of Health Boards) there shall be inserted the following paragraph—

"2A. In the case of a prescribed Health Board at least one of the persons appointed under paragraph 2 above must hold a post in a university with a medical or dental school."

3. In paragraph 4 of that Schedule (remuneration), after the words "Health Board" there shall be inserted "and to such other members of a Health Board as may be prescribed".

4. At the end of paragraph 5A of that Schedule there shall be added the words "and a direction under that paragraph may relate to a particular officer or servant or class of officer or servant specified in the direction".

5. After paragraph 7 of that Schedule there shall be inserted the following paragraphs—

"7A. Regulations may provide for the transfer of officers and servants from a Health Board to—

(a) another Health Board;

(b) the Agency; or

(c) a state hospital,

and for arrangements under which the services of an officer or servant of a Health Board are placed at the disposal of a body mentioned in sub-paragraphs (a) to (c).

7B. Directions may be given by the Secretary of State—

(a) to a Health Board to place services of any of its officers or servants at the disposal of a body mentioned in sub-paragraphs (a) to (c) of paragraph 7A; and

(b) to any such body to employ as an officer or servant any person who is or was employed by a Health Board and is specified in the direction,

and a Board or body to which such directions are given shall comply with the directions.

7C. Before making regulations under paragraph 7A or 8A, the Secretary of State shall consult such bodies and organisations as appear to him to be concerned."

6. After paragraph 8 of that Schedule there shall be inserted the following paragraph—

"8A. In connection with arrangements relating to community care services (within the meaning of section 5A(4) (local authority plans for community care services) of the Social Work (Scotland) Act 1968), regulations may make provision with respect to—

(a) the transfer to employment by a local authority of officers or servants employed by a Health Board; and

(b) the transfer to employment by a National Health Service body of officers and servants transferred to employment by a local authority by virtue of this paragraph,

and for the purposes of this paragraph "National Health Service body" means a Health Board, the Agency or an NHS trust.".

7. In paragraph 11(b) of that Schedule (delegation to committees etc), for the words "composed, as to a majority, by members of Health Boards" there shall be substituted "constituted in accordance with the regulations".

Common Services Agency

8. Schedule 5 to the 1978 Act shall be amended in accordance with paragraphs 9 to 12 below.

9. In paragraph 3 of that Schedule (appointment of chairman and members) for the words from "other members appointed" to the end there shall be substituted "such other members as the Secretary of State may, after consultation with the Health Boards, appoint."

10. In paragraph 3A of that Schedule (remuneration), after the words "management committee" there shall be inserted "and to such other members of the management committee as may be prescribed".

11. After paragraph 7A of that Schedule there shall be inserted the following paragraphs—

"7B. Regulations may provide for the transfer of officers and servants from the Agency to a Health Board or state hospital, and for arrangements under which the services of an officer or servant of the Agency are placed at the disposal of a Health Board or state hospital.

7C. Directions may be given by the Secretary of State—

(a) to the Agency to place services of any of its officers or servants at the disposal of a Health Board or state hospital; and

(b) to a Health Board or state hospital to employ as an officer or servant any person who is or was employed by the Agency and is specified in the direction,

and it shall be the duty of the Agency, a Health Board or a state hospital to comply with any such directions given to it."

12. After paragraph 8 of that Schedule there shall be inserted the following paragraphs—

"8A. In connection with arrangements relating to community care services (within the meaning of section 5A(4) (local authority plans for community care services) of the Social Work (Scotland) Act 1968), regulations may make provision with respect to—

(a) the transfer to employment by a local authority of officers or servants employed by the Agency; and

SCH. 5

(b) the transfer to employment by a National Health Service body of officers and servants transferred to employment by a local authority by virtue of this paragraph,

and for the purposes of this paragraph "National Health Service body" means the Agency, a Health Board or an NHS trust.

8B. Before making regulations under paragraph 7B or 8A, the Secretary of State shall consult such bodies and organisations as appear to him to be concerned.".

State hospitals

1984 c. 36.

13. In Schedule 1 to the Mental Health (Scotland) Act 1984 (State Hospital Management Committees)—

(a) in paragraph 6(b) (delegation to committees etc), for the words "composed, as to a majority, of members of a State Hospital Management Committee" there shall be substituted "constituted in accordance with the regulations"; and

(b) in paragraph 8 (application of provisions of the 1978 Act) the word "and" at the end of sub-paragraph (d) shall be omitted and after sub-paragraph (e) there shall be inserted—

"; and

(f) paragraphs 7A to 7C and 8A of Schedule 1 (which relate to the transfer of staff)."

Section 32.

SCHEDULE 6

SCHEDULES TO BE INSERTED AFTER SCHEDULE 7 TO THE NATIONAL HEALTH SERVICE (SCOTLAND) ACT 1978

"SCHEDULE 7A

NATIONAL HEALTH SERVICE TRUSTS

PART I

ORDERS ESTABLISHING NHS TRUSTS ETC.

1. Any reference in this Part of this Schedule to an order is a reference to an order under section 12A(1) establishing an NHS trust or any subsequent order under that provision amending or revoking a previous order.

2. The provisions made by an order shall be in conformity with any general provision made by regulations under section 12A(5).

3.—(1) Without prejudice to any amendment made by a subsequent order, the first order to be made in relation to any NHS trust shall specify—

(a) the name of the trust;

(b) the functions of the trust;

(c) the number of executive directors and non-executive directors;

(d) where the trust is to be regarded as having a significant teaching commitment, a provision to secure the inclusion in the non-executive directors referred to in paragraph (c) of a person appointed from a university with a medical or dental school specified in the order;

(e) the operational date of the trust, that is to say, the date on which the trust is to begin to undertake the whole of the functions conferred on it; and

(f) if a scheme is to be made under section 12B, the body (being a Health Board or the Agency) which is to make the scheme.

(2) For the purposes of sub-paragraph (1)(d), an NHS trust is to be regarded as having a significant teaching commitment in the following cases—

(a) if the trust is established to assume responsibility for the ownership and management of a hospital or other establishment or facility which, in the opinion of the Secretary of State, has a significant teaching and research commitment; and

(b) in any other case, if the Secretary of State so provides in the order.

(3) In a case where the order contains a provision made by virtue of sub-paragraph (1)(d) and a person who is being considered for appointment by virtue of that provision—

(a) is employed by the university in question; and

(b) would also, apart from this sub-paragraph, be regarded as employed by the trust,

his employment by the trust shall be disregarded in determining whether, if appointed, he will be a non-executive director of the trust.

(4) An order shall specify the accounting date of the trust.

4.—(1) An order may require a Health Board and the Agency to make staff, premises and other facilities available to an NHS trust pending the transfer or appointment of staff to or by the trust and the transfer of premises or other facilities to the trust.

(2) An order making provision under this paragraph may make provision with respect to the time when the Health Board's functions under the provision are to come to an end.

5.—(1) An order may provide for the establishment of an NHS trust with effect from a date earlier than the operational date of the trust and, during the period between that earlier date and the operational date, the trust shall have such limited functions for the purposes of enabling it to begin to operate satisfactorily with effect from the operational date as may be specified in the order.

(2) If an order makes the provision referred to in sub-paragraph (1), then, at any time during the period referred to in that sub-paragraph, the NHS trust shall be regarded as properly constituted (and may carry out its limited functions accordingly) notwithstanding that, at that time, all or any of the executive officers have not yet been appointed.

(3) If an order makes the provision referred to in sub-paragraph (1) above, the order may require a Health Board to discharge such liabilities of the NHS trust as—

(a) may be incurred during the period referred to in that sub-paragraph; and

(b) are of a description specified in the order.

Part II

Duties, Powers and Status of NHS Trusts

Specific duties

6.—(1) An NHS trust shall carry out effectively, efficiently and economically the functions for the time being conferred on it by an order under section 12A(1) and by the provisions of this Schedule and, with respect to the exercise of the powers conferred by an order under section 12A(8) or paragraphs 10 to 15, shall comply with any directions given to it by the Secretary of State, whether of a general or a particular nature.

SCH. 6

(2) An NHS trust shall comply with any directions given to it by the Secretary of State with respect to all or any of the following matters—

(a) the qualifications of persons who may be appointed as officers of the trust;

(b) the employment, for the purpose of performing functions specified in the direction, of officers having qualifications or experience of a description so specified;

(c) the manner in which officers of the trust are to be appointed;

(d) prohibiting or restricting the disposal of, or of any interest in, any asset which, at the time the direction is given, the Secretary of State reasonably considers to have a value in excess of such sum as may be specified in an order under section 12A(1) and in respect of which the Secretary of State considers that the interests of the National Health Service require that the asset should not be disposed of;

(e) compliance with guidance or directions given (by circular or otherwise) to Health Boards or particular descriptions of Health Boards, or the Agency; and

(f) the implementation of awards relating to the distinction or merit of medical practitioners or dental practitioners or any class or classes of such practitioners.

7.—(1) For each accounting year an NHS trust shall prepare and send to the Secretary of State an annual report in such form as may be determined by the Secretary of State.

(2) At such time or times as may be prescribed, an NHS trust shall hold a public meeting at which its audited accounts, its annual report, and such other documents as may be prèscribed shall be presented.

(3) In such circumstances and at such time or times as may be prescribed, an NHS trust shall hold a public meeting at which such documents as may be prescribed shall be presented.

8. An NHS trust shall furnish to the Secretary of State such reports, returns and other information, including information as to its forward planning as, and in such form as, he may require.

9.—(1) An NHS trust shall be liable to pay—

(a) to the chairman and any non-executive director of the trust—

(i) remuneration of an amount determined by the Secretary of State, not exceeding such amount as may be approved by the Treasury; and

(ii) such travelling and other allowances as may be determined by the Secretary of State with the approval of the Treasury; and

(b) to any member of a committee or sub-committee of the trust who is not also a director such travelling and other allowances as may be so determined.

(2) If an NHS trust so determines in the case of a person who is or has been a chairman of the trust, the trust shall be liable to pay such pension, allowances or gratuities to or in respect of him as may be determined by the Secretary of State with the approval of the Treasury.

(3) Different determinations may be made under sub-paragraph (1) or (2) in relation to different cases or description of cases.

Specific powers

10. An NHS trust may enter into NHS contracts.

SCH. 6

11. An NHS trust may undertake and commission research and make available staff and provide facilities for research by other persons.

12. An NHS trust may—

(a) provide training for persons employed or likely to be employed by the trust or otherwise in the provision of services under this Act; and

(b) make facilities and staff available in connection with training by a university or any other body providing training in connection with the health service.

13. An NHS trust may enter into arrangements for the carrying out, on such terms as seem to it to be appropriate, of any of its functions jointly with any Health Board, with the Agency, with another NHS trust or with any other body or individual.

14. According to the nature of its functions, an NHS trust may make accommodation or services or both available for patients who give undertakings (or for whom undertakings are given) to pay, in respect of the accommodation or services (or both) such charges as the trust may determine.

15. For the purpose of making additional income available in order better to perform its functions, an NHS trust shall have the powers specified in section 7(2) of the Health and Medicines Act 1988 (extension of powers of Secretary of State for financing the Health Service).

1988 c. 49.

General powers

16. Subject to Schedule 7B, an NHS trust shall have power to do anything which appears to it to be necessary or expedient for the purpose of or in connection with the discharge of its functions, including in particular power—

(a) to acquire and dispose of land and other property;

(b) to enter into such contracts as seem to the trust to be appropriate;

(c) to accept gifts of money, land or other property, including money, land or other property to be held on trust, for purposes relating to any service which it is their function to provide, administer, or make arrangements for, which purposes shall include any purposes relating to a hospital or other establishment or facility which is provided or managed by the trust; and

(d) to employ staff on such terms as the trust thinks fit.

17. In connection with arrangements relating to community care services (within the meaning of section 5A(4) (local authority plans for community care services) of the Social Work (Scotland) Act 1968), the Secretary of State may by regulations make provision with respect to—

(a) the transfer to employment by a local authority of staff employed by an NHS trust; and

(b) the transfer to employment by a National Health Service body of staff transferred to employment by a local authority by virtue of this paragraph,

and for the purposes of this paragraph "National Health Service body" means an NHS trust, a Health Board or the Agency.

18. Regulations made under paragraph 17 may make such incidental and consequential provision in relation to staff transferred by virtue of that paragraph as may be made in relation to officers and servants of a Health Board transferred by virtue of regulations made under paragraph 8A of Schedule 1.

SCH. 6

19. Before making regulations under paragraph 17, the Secretary of State shall consult such bodies and organisations as appear to him to be concerned.

20.—(1) Without prejudice to the generality of paragraph 16, to or in respect of such of its employees as it may determine, an NHS trust may make such arrangements for providing pensions, allowances or gratuities as it may determine; and such arrangements may include the establishment and administration, by the trust or otherwise, of one or more pension schemes.

(2) The reference in sub-paragraph (1) to pensions, allowances or gratuities to or in respect of employees of an NHS trust includes a reference to pensions, allowances or gratuities by way of compensation to or in respect of any of the trust's employees who suffer loss of office or employment or loss or diminution of emoluments.

Status

21. An NHS trust shall not be regarded as the servant or agent of the Crown or, except as provided by this Act, as enjoying any status, immunity or privilege of the Crown; and an NHS trust's property shall not be regarded as property of, or property held on behalf of, the Crown.

PART III

SUPPLEMENTARY PROVISIONS

Reimbursement for health services work carried out otherwise than under contract

22.—(1) In any case where an NHS trust provides goods or services for the benefit of an individual and—

(a) those goods or services are not provided pursuant to an NHS contract; and

(b) the condition of the individual is such that he needs those goods or services and, having regard to his condition, it is not practicable before providing them to enter into an NHS contract for their provision, and

(c) the provision of those goods or services is a function of a Health Board or is within the primary functions of a District Health Authority within the meaning of the National Health Service Act 1977,

the trust shall be remunerated by that Board or Authority in respect of the provision of the goods or services in question.

(2) The rate of any remuneration payable by virtue of sub-paragraph (1) shall be calculated in such manner or on such basis as may be determined by the Secretary of State.

23. In any case where an NHS trust provides goods or services for the benefit of an individual and—

(a) paragraph 22(1)(a) applies but paragraph 22(1)(c) does not apply; and

(b) the individual is resident outside the United Kingdom and is of a description (being a description associating the individual with another country) specified for the purposes of this paragraph by a direction made by the Secretary of State,

the trust shall be remunerated by the Secretary of State in respect of the provision of the goods or services in question at such rate or rates as he considers appropriate.

Use and development of land used for religious purposes and burial grounds

SCH. 6

24. Where land consisting of a church or other building used or formerly used for religious worship, or the site thereof, or a burial ground, within the meaning of section 118 of the Town and Country Planning (Scotland) Act 1972 (provisions as to churches and burial grounds), is held by an NHS trust for any of its purposes, that section applies to the land as if—

1972 c. 52.

(a) the land had been acquired by the trust as mentioned in subsection (1) of that section; and

(b) the trust were a statutory undertaker, within the meaning of that Act.

PART IV

DISSOLUTION

25.—(1) The Secretary of State may by order dissolve an NHS trust.

(2) An order under this paragraph may be made—

(a) on the application of the NHS trust concerned; or

(b) if the Secretary of State considers it appropriate in the interests of the health service as a whole.

(3) Except where it appears to the Secretary of State necessary to make an order under this paragraph as a matter of urgency, no such order shall be made until after the completion of such consultation as may be prescribed.

26.—(1) If an NHS trust is dissolved under this Part of this Schedule, the Secretary of State may by order transfer or provide for the transfer to—

(a) the Secretary of State, or

(b) a Health Board, or

(c) the Agency, or

(d) another NHS trust,

of such of the property, rights and liabilities of the NHS trust which is dissolved as in his opinion is appropriate and any such order may include provisions corresponding to those of section 12D.

(2) An order under this paragraph may make provision in connection with the transfer of staff employed by or for the purposes of the NHS trust which is dissolved; and such an order may include provisions corresponding to those of sections 12B and 12C, including provision for the making of a scheme by such body (being a Health Board or the Agency) as may be specified in the order.

(3) No order shall be made under this paragraph until after completion of such consultation as may be prescribed.

27. If an NHS trust is dissolved under this Part of this Schedule, the Secretary of State or such other NHS trust or Health Board as he may direct or, if he so directs, the Agency shall undertake the responsibility for the continued payment of any such pension, allowances or gratuities as, by virtue of paragraph 9(2) or paragraph 20 above, would otherwise have been the responsibility of the trust which has been dissolved.

28. An NHS trust may not be dissolved or wound up except in accordance with this Part of this Schedule.

SCH. 6

SCHEDULE 7B

FINANCIAL PROVISIONS RELATING TO NHS TRUSTS

Borrowing

1.—(1) Subject to the provisions of this paragraph and to any limit imposed under the following provisions of this Schedule, for the purpose of its functions an NHS trust may borrow (both temporarily, by way of overdraft, and longer term) from the Secretary of State or from any other person.

(2) An NHS trust may not grant any security over any of its assets or in any other way use any of its assets as security for a loan.

(3) Except with the consent of the Secretary of State, an NHS trust may not borrow in any currency other than sterling; and the Secretary of State shall not give his consent to any such borrowing except with the approval of the Treasury.

(4) Interest on any sums borrowed from the Secretary of State by an NHS trust shall be paid at such variable or fixed rates and at such times as the Treasury may determine.

(5) A rate of interest under sub-paragraph (4) shall be determined as if section 5 of the National Loans Act 1968 had effect in respect of it and subsections (5) to (5B) of that section shall apply accordingly.

1968 c. 13.

(6) Subject to sub-paragraphs (4) and (5), the terms on which any sums are borrowed from the Secretary of State by an NHS trust shall be such as he may determine; and, in the event of the early repayment of any sums so borrowed, such terms may require the payment of a premium or allow a discount.

Guarantees of borrowing

2.—(1) The Secretary of State may guarantee, in such manner and on such conditions as, with the approval of the Treasury, he considers appropriate, the repayments of the principal of and the payment of interest on any sums which an NHS trust borrows from a person other than the Secretary of State.

(2) Immediately after a guarantee is given under this paragraph, the Secretary of State shall lay a statement of the guarantee before each House of Parliament.

(3) Where any sum is issued for fulfilling a guarantee so given, the Secretary of State shall lay before each House of Parliament a statement relating to that sum as soon as possible after the end of each financial year beginning with that in which the sum is issued and ending with that in which all liability in respect of the principal of the sum and in respect of interest on it is finally discharged.

(4) If any sums are issued in fulfilment of a guarantee given under this paragraph, the NHS trust concerned shall make to the Secretary of State, at such times and in such manner as the Secretary of State may from time to time direct,—

(a) payments of such amounts as the Secretary of State with the consent of the Treasury so directs in or towards repayment of the sums so issued; and

(b) payments of interest, at such rates as the Secretary of State with the consent of the Treasury so directs, on what is outstanding for the time being in respect of sums so issued.

Limits on indebtedness

3.—(1) The aggregate of all sums borrowed by NHS trusts established to assume responsibility for the ownership and management of, or to provide and manage, hospitals or other establishments or facilities which are situated in Scotland shall not exceed £500 million or such other sum not exceeding £1,000 million as may be specified by order made by the Secretary of State with the consent of the Treasury.

(2) The reference in sub-paragraph (1) to sums borrowed does not include a reference to the initial loan of NHS trusts.

4. Any power to make an order under paragraph 3 shall be exercisable by statutory instrument which shall be subject to annulment in pursuance of a resolution of the House of Commons.

Additional public dividend capital

5.—(1) If the Secretary of State, with the consent of the Treasury, considers it appropriate to do so, he may, instead of making a loan to an NHS trust under paragraph 1, pay an amount to the trust as public dividend capital.

(2) Section 12E shall apply to public dividend capital paid to an NHS trust under this paragraph as it applies to public dividend capital forming part of the trust's originating capital debt.

Surplus funds

6. If it appears to the Secretary of State that any amount standing in the reserves of an NHS trust is surplus to its foreseeable requirements, the trust shall, if the Secretary of State with the approval of the Treasury and after consultation with the trust so directs, pay that amount into the Consolidated Fund.

Investment

7. An NHS trust may not invest any money held by it except in securities of the Government of the United Kingdom or in such other manner as the Secretary of State may with the consent of the Treasury approve."

SCHEDULE 7

Section 36.

Amendments relating to Audit of Accounts of Scottish Health Service Bodies

The Local Government (Scotland) Act 1973

1. Part VII of the Local Government (Scotland) Act 1973 (finance) shall be amended in accordance with paragraphs 2 to 13 below.

1973 c. 65.

2. In section 96 (accounts and audit of local authorities), in subsection (4), for the words "Commission for Local Authority Accounts" there shall be substituted "Accounts Commission for Scotland".

3.—(1) Section 97 (establishment of Commission for Local Authority Accounts in Scotland) shall be amended as follows.

(2) In subsection (1)—

(a) for the words "Commission for Local Authority Accounts in Scotland" there shall be substituted "Accounts Commission for Scotland";

(b) for the word "twelve" there shall be substituted "fifteen";

(c) for the word "nine" there shall be substituted "eleven"; and

(d) after the word "authorities" there shall be inserted "and such organisations connected with the health service".

(3) In subsection (2)—

(a) in paragraph (a)—

(i) after the words "accounts of" there shall be inserted "(i)", and

(ii) after the word "authorities" there shall be inserted the following sub-paragraphs—

"(ii) the bodies mentioned in section 86(1)(a) to (c) of the National Health Service (Scotland) Act 1978;

SCH 7

(iii) the members of every recognised fund-holding practice;

(iv) the Mental Welfare Commission for Scotland; and

(v) any State Hospital Management Committee constituted under section 91 of the Mental Health (Scotland) Act 1984,";

(b) in paragraph (c), after the word "authorities" there shall be inserted "or, as the case may be, health service bodies"; and

(c) in paragraph (d), after the word "authorities" there shall be inserted "or health service bodies".

(4) After subsection (2) there shall be inserted the following subsections—

"(2A) Subject to section 100(1A) of this Act, in relation to the members of a recognised fund-holding practice, any reference in this Part of this Act to their accounts is a reference only to the accounts relating to allotted sums paid to them.

(2B) In this Part of this Act—

"health service body" means a body referred to in subsection (2)(a)(ii) to (v) above; and

"recognised fund-holding practice" and "allotted sum" have the same meanings as in section 87B of the National Health Service (Scotland) Act 1978."

(5) In subsection (3), after the word "authorities" there shall be inserted "and such organisations connected with the health service".

(6) After subsection (4) there shall be inserted the following subsections—

"(4A) It shall be the duty of the Commission to make, by such date as the Secretary of State may determine, an offer of employment by the Commission to each person employed in the civil service of the State in connection with the audit of the accounts of any health service body whose name is notified to the Commission by the Secretary of State for the purposes of this subsection; and the terms of the offer must be such that they are, taken as a whole, not less favourable to the person to whom the offer is made than the terms on which he is employed on the date on which the offer is made.

(4B) An offer made in pursuance of subsection (4A) above shall not be revocable during the period of three months beginning with the date on which it is made.

(4C) Where a person becomes an officer of the Commission in consequence of subsection (4A) above, then, for the purposes of the Employment Protection (Consolidation) Act 1978, his period of employment in the civil service of the State shall count as a period of employment by the Commission and the change of employment shall not break the continuity of the period of employment.

(4D) Where a person ceases to be employed as mentioned in subsection (4A) above—

(a) on becoming an officer of the Commission in consequence of an offer made in pursuance of that subsection; or

(b) having unreasonably refused such an offer,

he shall not, on ceasing to be so employed, be treated for the purposes of any scheme under section 1 of the Superannuation Act 1972 as having been retired on redundancy."

(7) At the end of subsection (6) there shall be added—

"or a person who is, within the period of five years beginning with the relevant date, approved by the Secretary of State, acting on the recommendation of the Commission and whose approval is not (whether during that period or after its expiry) withdrawn by the Secretary of State acting on such recommendation.

(6A) In subsection (6) above, "the relevant date" means the date appointed for the coming into force of paragraph 3(3) of Schedule 7 to the National Health Service and Community Care Act 1990."

4.—(1) Section 97A (studies for improving economy etc in services) shall be amended as follows.

(2) At the end of subsection (2) there shall be added "and, in the case of studies relating to a health service body, shall, on request, furnish to the Comptroller and Auditor General all material relevant to the studies."

(3) At the end of subsection (3) there shall be added "and, in the case of a health service body, the Commission shall also consult the Secretary of State and the Comptroller and Auditor General."

5.—(1) Section 98 (expenses and accounts of Commission) shall be amended as follows.

(2) In subsection (1)—

(a) in paragraph (b), after the word "Commission" where it first occurs there shall be inserted "relating to their functions with respect to local authorities"; and

(b) at the end of paragraph (b) there shall be inserted the following paragraph—

"(c) such part of the expenses of the Commission relating to their functions with respect to health service bodies as is not met by grants under paragraph (a) above shall be met by health service bodies in accordance with regulations made by the Secretary of State after consultation with such organisations connected with the health service as appear to him to be concerned."

(3) In subsection (2), after "(b)" there shall be inserted "or (c)".

6. In section 99 (general duties of auditors)—

(a) after the word "authority" in both places where it occurs there shall be inserted "or health service body"; and

(b) in paragraph (a), after the word "Act" there shall be inserted "or, in the case of a health service body, directions under section 86(3) of the National Health Service (Scotland) Act 1978".

7.—(1) Section 100 (auditor's right of access to documents) shall be amended as follows.

(2) In subsection (1)—

(a) after the word "authority" where it first occurs there shall be inserted "or health service body"; and

(b) after the word "authority" in the second place where it occurs there shall be inserted "or body".

(3) After subsection (1) there shall be inserted the following subsection—

"(1A) In the case of a recognised fund-holding practice, the reference in subsection (1) above to documents includes a reference to documents relating to all the accounts and records of the members of the practice, whether or not relating to an allotted sum."

SCH 7

(4) In subsection (2), after the word "authority" there shall be inserted "and health service body".

8. In section 101 (completion of audit), after subsection (4) there shall be added the following subsection—

"(5) Within 14 days of the completion of the audit of the accounts of a health service body the auditor shall place on any abstract of those accounts prepared by the health service body by virtue of section 86 of the National Health Service (Scotland) Act 1978 a certificate, in such form as the Commission may direct, to the effect that he has audited the accounts in accordance with the provisions of this Part of this Act; and the auditor shall, on so certifying, forthwith send copies of the abstract of the accounts to the Commission, the Secretary of State and the health service body."

9.—(1) Section 102 (reports to Commission by Controller of Audit) shall be amended as follows.

(2) In subsection (1)—

(a) after the word "authorities" there shall be inserted "and health service bodies"; and

(b) after the word "authority" there shall be inserted "or health service body".

(3) After subsection (4) there shall be added the following subsection—

"(5) Without prejudice to subsection (1) above and section 104A(2) of this Act, the Controller of Audit may make a report to the Commission on any matters arising out of or in connection with the accounts of a health service body and shall send a copy of any report so made to any health service body which is named in that report and to the Secretary of State."

10. In section 103 (action by Commission on reports by Controller of Audit), after the word "Audit" there shall be inserted "with respect to the accounts of any local authority".

11. After section 104 there shall be inserted the following section—

"Audit of accounts of health service bodies: special provisions.

104A.—(1) Where the auditor of the accounts of a health service body has reason to believe that the body, or any officer of the body—

(a) has made a decision which involves the incurring of expenditure which is unlawful; or

(b) has taken a course of action which, if pursued to its conclusion, would be unlawful and likely to cause a loss or deficiency,

he shall forthwith make a report to the Controller of Audit.

(2) On receipt of a report under subsection (1) above the Controller of Audit—

(a) shall forthwith send a copy of the report to the Commission and to the Secretary of State; and

(b) may, if he thinks fit, send to the Commission and to the Secretary of State any observations which he may have on the report.

(3) The Commission may make a report to the Secretary of State on any matters arising out of or in connection with the accounts of a health service body."

12. After subsection (2) of section 106 (application of sections 93 to 105 to bodies other than local authorities and to officers) there shall be added the following subsection—

"(3) In the application of subsection (2) above to an officer of a health service body, for the words from "96" to "section 105" there shall be substituted "97 to 104A."."

13. In Schedule 8 (provisions as to the Commission), for the words "Commission for Local Authority Accounts in Scotland" in both places where they occur there shall be substituted "Accounts Commission for Scotland".

The National Health Service (Scotland) Act 1978

14.—(1) Section 86 of the National Health Service (Scotland) Act 1978 (keeping and audit of accounts of certain Scottish health bodies) shall be amended as follows.

1978 c. 29.

(2) In subsections (1) and (1A), for the words "by auditors appointed by the Secretary of State" there shall be substituted "in accordance with Part VII of the Local Government (Scotland) Act 1973 by auditors appointed by the Accounts Commission for Scotland".

(3) After subsection (1B) there shall be inserted the following subsection—

"(1C) In such circumstances and to such extent as regulations made by the Secretary of State so provide, the requirement in subsection (1A)(a) to have accounts audited shall not apply to the accounts for any year of a recognised fund-holding practice if those accounts are submitted to a Health Board and summarised in the Board's accounts."

(4) Subsection (2) shall cease to have effect.

General amendment

15. Without prejudice to any express amendment made by this Act, for any reference in any enactment (including an enactment comprised in subordinate legislation) to the Commission for Local Authority Accounts in Scotland there shall be substituted a reference to the Accounts Commission for Scotland.

SCHEDULE 8

Section 60.

PROVISIONS ARISING OUT OF REMOVAL OF CROWN IMMUNITIES FROM HEALTH SERVICE BODIES

PART I

AMENDMENTS CONTINUING CERTAIN STATUTORY EXEMPTIONS

The Employers' Liability (Compulsory Insurance) Act 1969

1. In section 3 of the Employers' Liability (Compulsory Insurance) Act 1969 (employers exempted from insurance), in subsection (2) after the words "subsection (1)(a) above" there shall be inserted—

1969 c. 57.

"(a) a health service body, as defined in section 60(7) of the National Health Service and Community Care Act 1990, and a National Health Service trust established under Part I of that Act or the National Health Service (Scotland) Act 1978; and

(b)".

The Vehicles (Excise) Act 1971

2. In section 7 of the Vehicles (Excise) Act 1971 (miscellaneous exemptions from duty), after subsection (4) there shall be inserted the following subsection—

1971 c. 10.

SCH. 8

"(4A) A mechanically propelled vehicle shall not be chargeable with any duty under this Act at a time when it is used or kept on a road by a health service body, as defined in section 60(7) of the National Health Service and Community Care Act 1990 or a National Health Service trust established under Part I of that Act or the National Health Service (Scotland) Act 1978."

1978 c. 29.

The Copyright, Designs and Patents Act 1988

1988 c. 48.

3. At the end of section 48 of the Copyright, Designs and Patents Act 1988 (material communicated to the Crown in the course of public business) there shall be added the following subsection—

"(6) In this section "the Crown" includes a health service body, as defined in section 60(7) of the National Health Service and Community Care Act 1990, and a National Health Service trust established under Part I of that Act or the National Health Service (Scotland) Act 1978; and the reference in subsection (1) above to public business shall be construed accordingly."

The Road Traffic Act 1988

1988 c. 52.

4. In section 144 of the Road Traffic Act 1988 (exceptions from requirement of third-party insurance or security) in subsection (2) after paragraph (d) there shall be inserted the following paragraphs—

"(da) to a vehicle owned by a health service body, as defined in section 60(7) of the National Health Service and Community Care Act 1990, at a time when the vehicle is being driven under the owner's control,

(db) to an ambulance owned by a National Health Service trust established under Part I of the National Health Service and Community Care Act 1990 or the National Health Service (Scotland) Act 1978, at a time when a vehicle is being driven under the owner's control".

PART II
CONSEQUENTIAL AMENDMENTS

The Acquisition of Land (Authorisation Procedure) (Scotland) Act 1947

1947 c. 42.

5. In the First Schedule to the Acquisition of Land (Authorisation Procedure) (Scotland) Act 1947 (procedure for authorising compulsory purchases), after paragraph 10 there shall be inserted the following paragraph—

"10A. In paragraphs 9 and 10 of this Schedule "statutory undertakers" include—

(a) a health service body, as defined in section 60(7) of the National Health Service and Community Care Act 1990; and

(b) a National Health Service trust established under Part I of that Act or the National Health Service (Scotland) Act 1978;

but in relation to a health service body, as so defined, any reference in those paragraphs to land acquired or available for acquisition by the statutory undertakers shall be construed as a reference to land acquired or available for use by the Secretary of State for use or occupation by that body."

The Town and Country Planning Act 1971

SCH. 8

6. In section 128 of the Town and Country Planning Act 1971 (use and development of consecrated land and burial grounds) after subsection (4) there shall be inserted the following subsection—

1971 c. 78.

"(4A) In the case of land—

(a) which has been acquired by the Secretary of State under subsection (1) of section 87 of the National Health Service Act 1977 or to which, by virtue of subsection (6) of that section, this section applies as if it had been so acquired, and

(b) which is held, used or occupied by a health service body, as defined in section 60(7) of the National Health Service and Community Care Act 1990,

subsection (1) or, as the case may be, subsection (4) above shall apply with the omission of paragraph (a) and, in paragraph (b), of the words "in any other case"."

The Town and Country Planning (Scotland) Act 1972

7. In section 118 of the Town and Country Planning (Scotland) Act 1972 (provisions as to churches and burial grounds), after subsection (1) there shall be inserted the following subsection—

1972 c. 52.

"(1A) In the case of land—

(a) which has been acquired by the Secretary of State under section 79(1) of the National Health Service (Scotland) Act 1978; and

(b) which is held, used or occupied by a health service body, as defined in section 60(7) of the National Health Service and Community Care Act 1990),

subsection (1) of this section shall apply with the omission of paragraph (a) and, in paragraph (b), of the words "in any other case"."

The Acquisition of Land Act 1981

8.—(1) At the end of section 16 of the Acquisition of Land Act 1981 (statutory undertakers' land excluded from compulsory purchase) there shall be added the following subsection—

1981 c. 67.

"(3) In the preceding provisions of this section "statutory undertakers" include—

(a) a health service body, as defined in section 60(7) of the National Health Service and Community Care Act 1990; and

(b) a National Health Service trust established under Part I of that Act or the National Health Service (Scotland) Act 1978;

but in relation to a health service body, as so defined, any reference in those provisions to land acquired or available for acquisition by the statutory undertakers shall be construed as a reference to land acquired or available for acquisition by the Secretary of State for use or occupation by that body".

(2) In section 17 of that Act (local authority and statutory undertakers' land) at the end of subsection (2) there shall be inserted the following subsection—

"(2A) Subsection (3) of section 16 above applies in relation to subsections (1) and (2) above as it applies in relation to the preceding provisions of that section."

SCH. 8

The Value Added Tax Act 1983

1983 c. 55.

9. In section 27 of the Value Added Tax Act 1983 (application to Crown), in subsection (4) after the words "Minister of the Crown" there shall be inserted the words "including a health service body, as defined in section 60(7) of the National Health Service and Community Care Act 1990".

The Housing Act 1988

1988 c. 50.

10. In Schedule 2 to the Housing Act 1988 (grounds for possession of dwelling-houses let on assured tenancies), at the end of Ground 16 (dwelling-house let in consequence of employment by the landlord) there shall be added the following paragraph—

"For the purposes of this ground, at a time when the landlord is or was the Secretary of State, employment by a health service body, as defined in section 60(7) of the National Health Service and Community Care Act 1990, shall be regarded as employment by the Secretary of State."

The Housing (Scotland) Act 1988

1988 c. 43.

11. In Schedule 5 to the Housing (Scotland) Act 1988 (grounds for possession of houses let on assured tenancies) at the end of Ground 17 (house let in consequence of employment by the landlord) there shall be added the following paragraph—

"For the purposes of this ground, at a time when the landlord is or was the Secretary of State, employment by a health service body, as defined in section 60(7) of the National Health Service and Community Care Act 1990, shall be regarded as employment by the Secretary of State."

PART III
TRANSITIONAL PROVISIONS

12. In this Part of this Schedule—

(a) "the appointed day" means the day appointed for the coming into force of subsection (1) of section 60 of this Act;

(b) "functional health service land" means land which for the time being falls within paragraph (a) or paragraph (b) of that subsection;

(c) "health service body" has the same meaning as in that section; and

(d) "NHS trust" means such a trust established under Part I of this Act or the National Health Service (Scotland) Act 1978.

1978 c. 29.

The Building (Scotland) Act 1959

13.—(1) Notwithstanding section 60(1) of this Act, where, on or after the appointed day, relevant work is carried out by or on behalf of a health service body or an NHS trust—

(a) in relation to a building which is, immediately before the appointed day, a Crown building within the meaning of section 26(3) of the Building (Scotland) Act 1959 (application to the Crown); or

1959 c. 24.

(b) in constructing a building which, if it had been constructed before the appointed day, would have been a Crown building within the meaning of that provision,

Part II of that Act shall apply to the relevant work as if it were being carried out before the appointed day.

(2) In sub-paragraph (1) above, "relevant work" means work in respect of which, before the appointed day, a health service body has granted a certificate that the detail design has been completed.

The Medicines Act 1968

Sch. 8

14.—(1) In any case where—

(a) before the appointed day, a health service body or an NHS trust has made an application for a licence under Part II of the Medicines Act 1968 or any such application as is referred to in section 36 of that Act (applications for clinical trial and animal test certificates), and

1968 c. 67.

(b) the application was accompanied by a declaration under paragraph (a) or paragraph (b) of sub-paragraph (2) below, and

(c) the application has not been determined before the appointed day,

then, on and after the appointed day and until the application is determined, the health service body or NHS trust concerned shall be treated for all purposes as if it held a licence or, as the case may be, a certificate of the description applied for.

(2) The declarations referred to in sub-paragraph (1)(b) above are,—

(a) in the case of a health service body, that, at the date of the application, the body was carrying on activities which, after the appointed day, it would be unlawful to carry on except in accordance with a licence or certificate of the description applied for; and

(b) in the case of an NHS trust, that the trust has been established to assume responsibility for the ownership and management of a hospital or other establishment or facility and, at the date of the application, a health service body was carrying on at that hospital, establishment or facility activities which it is unlawful for the NHS trust to carry on except in accordance with a licence or certificate of the description applied for.

(3) For the purposes of sub-paragraph (1) above, an application is determined when the licensing authority—

(a) grant a licence or, as the case may be, certificate to the applicant (whether or not in accordance with the application); or

(b) notify the applicant of their refusal to grant a licence or certificate on the application.

(4) Expressions used in sub-paragraphs (1) to (3) above have the same meaning as in sections 18 to 22 of the Medicines Act 1968 (applications for, and grant of, licences), including, where applicable, any of those sections as applied by subsection (3) of section 36 of that Act in relation to applications falling within subsection (1) of that section.

The Fire Precautions Act 1971

15.—(1) Without prejudice to the continuing validity on and after the appointed day of any fire certificate issued before that day in accordance with subsection (3) of section 40 of the Fire Precautions Act 1971 (certain functions in relation to premises occupied or owned by the Crown exercisable by a fire inspector instead of by the fire authority), any application made, notice issued or other thing done before the appointed day to or by a fire inspector in relation to premises held, used or occupied by a health service body, shall be treated on and after that day as if made, issued or done to or by a fire authority.

1971 c. 40.

(2) Expressions used in sub-paragraph (1) above have the same meaning as in the Fire Precautions Act 1971.

The Town and Country Planning Act 1971

16.—(1) This paragraph applies if—

(a) before the appointed day, notice of any proposed development has been given to a local planning authority in accordance with arrangements relating to development by government departments; and

SCH. 8

(b) the development relates to land which, at the time the notice was given, was functional health service land; and

(c) the proposed development has not been carried out before the appointed day.

(2) So far as relates to the carrying out of the development of which notice was given as mentioned in sub-paragraph (1)(a) above, for the purposes of the arrangements referred to in that paragraph and of the Town and Country Planning Act 1971,—

1971 c. 78.

(a) the carrying out of the development shall continue to be regarded as being by or on behalf of the Crown; and

(b) so long as the interest of the Secretary of State in the land referred to in sub-paragraph (1)(b) above continues on and after the appointed day to be held in fact by the Secretary of State or an NHS trust, that interest shall be regarded as continuing to be an interest of, or held on behalf of, the Crown.

(3) Subject to paragraph 12 above, expressions used in sub-paragraphs (1) and (2) above have the same meaning as in the Town and Country Planning Act 1971.

The Town and Country Planning (Scotland) Act 1972

17.—(1) This paragraph applies if—

(a) before the appointed day, notice of any proposed development has been given to a planning authority in accordance with arrangements relating to development by government departments; and

(b) the development relates to land which, at the time the notice was given, was functional health service land; and

(c) the proposed development has not been carried out before the appointed day.

(2) So far as relates to the carrying out of the development of which notice was given as mentioned in sub-paragraph (1)(a) above, for the purposes of the arrangements referred to in that paragraph and of the Town and Country Planning (Scotland) Act 1972—

1972 c. 52.

(a) the carrying out of the development shall continue to be regarded as being by or on behalf of the Crown; and

(b) so long as the interest of the Secretary of State in the land referred to in sub-paragraph (1)(b) above continues on and after the appointed day to be held in fact by the Secretary of State or an NHS trust, that interest shall be regarded as continuing to be an interest of, or held on behalf of, the Crown.

(3) Subject to paragraph 12 above, expressions used in sub-paragraphs (1) and (2) above have the same meaning as in the Town and Country Planning (Scotland) Act 1972.

The Building Act 1984

18.—(1) If, immediately before the appointed day, approved work is proposed to be carried out by or on behalf of a Crown authority (whether or not in relation to a Crown building) the fact that, on or after the appointed day, the work may be carried out by or on behalf of a health service body or an NHS trust shall not prevent it continuing to be regarded for the purposes of Part I of the Building Act 1984 as work carried out by a Crown authority.

1984 c. 55.

(2) Subject to sub-paragraph (3) below, expressions used in sub-paragraph (1) above have the same meaning as in section 44 of the Building Act 1984 (application of Part I to Crown).

1984 c. 55.

(3) Any reference in sub-paragraph (1) above to approved work is a reference to work in respect of which, before the appointed day, either a contract for carrying it out was entered into or all necessary design certificates were signed in accordance with arrangements relating to compliance with the substantive requirements of building regulations by Regional and District Health Authorities and certain Special Health Authorities.

The Housing Act 1988 and the Rent Act 1977

19.—(1) This paragraph applies to a tenancy—

(a) which was entered into before the appointed day; and

(b) which is of land in England or Wales which, immediately before the appointed day, was functional health service land.

(2) If and so long as the interest of the landlord under a tenancy to which this paragraph applies continues on and after the appointed day to belong in fact either to the Secretary of State or to an NHS trust, it shall be taken to belong to a government department for the purposes of—

(a) paragraph 11 of Schedule 1 to the Housing Act 1988 (Crown tenancies entered into after the commencement of Part I of that Act not to be assured tenancies); or

1988 c. 50.

(b) section 13 of the Rent Act 1977 (earlier Crown tenancies not to be protected tenancies).

1977 c. 42.

(3) Expressions used in sub-paragraphs (1) and (2) above have the same meaning as in Part I of the Housing Act 1988 or, as the case may require, the Rent Act 1977.

The Housing (Scotland) Act 1988 and the Rent (Scotland) Act 1984

20.—(1) This paragraph applies to a tenancy—

(a) which was entered into before the appointed day; and

(b) which is of land in Scotland which, immediately before the appointed day, was functional health service land.

(2) If and so long as the interest of the landlord under a tenancy to which this paragraph applies continues on and after the appointed day to belong in fact either to the Secretary of State or to an NHS trust, it shall be taken to belong to a government department for the purposes of—

(a) paragraph 10 of Schedule 4 to the Housing (Scotland) Act 1988 (Crown tenancies entered into after the commencement of that Schedule not to be assured tenancies); or

1988 c. 43.

(b) section 4 of the Rent (Scotland) Act 1984 (earlier Crown tenancies not to be protected tenancies).

1984 c. 58.

(3) Expressions used in sub-paragraphs (1) and (2) above have the same meaning as in Part II of the Housing (Scotland) Act 1988 or, as the case may be, the Rent (Scotland) Act 1984.

SCHEDULE 9

Section 66(1).

Minor and Consequential Amendments

The Public Health (Scotland) Act 1897

1897 c. 38.

1.—(1) In section 54 of the Public Health (Scotland) Act 1897 (removal of infected persons without proper lodging to hospital), after the words "Secretary of State" in both places where they occur, there shall be inserted the words "or to any hospital managed by a National Health Service trust established under section 12A of the National Health Service (Scotland) Act 1978".

(2) In section 55(1) of that Act (detention of infected persons without proper lodging in hospital) after the word "hospital", where it first appears, there shall be inserted the words "vested in the Secretary of State or managed by a National Health Service trust established under section 12A of the National Health Service (Scotland) Act 1978".

(3) In section 55(3) of that Act, after the words "vested in the Secretary of State" there shall be inserted the words "or managed by a National Health Service trust established under section 12A of the National Health Service (Scotland) Act 1978".

(4) In section 96 of that Act (power of local authority to remove sick persons to hospital), after the words "Secretary of State" there shall be inserted the words "or managed by a National Health Service trust established under section 12A of the National Health Service (Scotland) Act 1978".

The Voluntary Hospitals (Paying Patients) Act 1936

1936 c. 17.

2. In section 1 of the Voluntary Hospitals (Paying Patients) Act 1936 (definitions)—

(a) in the definition of "voluntary hospital", after the words "of the rates" there shall be inserted "or which is vested in an NHS trust"; and

(b) after the definition of "committee of management" there shall be inserted—

""NHS trust" means a National Health Service trust established under Part I of the National Health Service and Community Care Act 1990."

The Nursing Homes Registration (Scotland) Act 1938

1938 c. 73.

3. In section 10(3)(a) (interpretation) of the Nursing Homes Registration (Scotland) Act 1938, after the words "local authority" there shall be inserted the words "or a National Health Service trust established under section 12A of the National Health Service (Scotland) Act 1978.".

The Public Health (Scotland) Act 1945

1945 c. 15. (9 & 10 Geo. 6).

4. In section 1(3) of the Public Health (Scotland) Act 1945 (regulations with regard to treatment and prevention of spread of certain diseases)—

(a) after the words "Health Boards" there shall be inserted the words "or National Health Service trusts established under section 12A of the National Health Service (Scotland) Act 1978"; and

(b) in the proviso to that subsection, after the word "Board" there shall be inserted the words "National Health Service trust,".

The National Assistance Act 1948

1948 c. 29.

5.—(1) At the beginning of subsection (4) of section 21 of the National Assistance Act 1948 (accommodation provided under section 21 to be provided in premises managed by a local authority) there shall be inserted "Subject to the provisions of section 26 of this Act".

(2) For paragraphs (b) and (c) of subsection (7) of that section (which enable health services to be provided on premises where accommodation is provided under that section) there shall be substituted—

"(b) make arrangements for the provision on the premises in which the accommodation is being provided of such other services as appear to the authority to be required."

(3) At the end of subsection (8) of that section (which excludes from that section provision required to be made by a local authority under other enactments) there shall be inserted "or authorised or required to be provided under the National Health Service Act 1977".

(4) In section 24 of that Act (authority liable for provision of accommodation)—

(a) in subsection (6) for the words from "patient" to "shall" there shall be substituted "patient in a hospital vested in the Secretary of State or an NHS trust shall"; and

(b) at the end there shall be added—

"(7) In subsection (6) above "NHS trust" means a National Health Service trust established under Part I of the National Health Service and Community Care Act 1990 or under the National Health Service (Scotland) Act 1978."

(5) In section 26 of that Act (provision of accommodation in premises maintained by voluntary organisations etc.)—

(a) in subsection (2) the words "subsection (1) of" shall be omitted;

(b) after subsection (4) there shall be inserted—

"(4A) Section 21(5) of this Act shall have effect as respects accommodation provided under arrangements made by virtue of this section with the substitution for the reference to the authority managing the premises of a reference to the authority making the arrangements.";

(c) in subsection (5) the words "subsection (1) of" shall be omitted.

(6) Subsections (2) and (3) of section 35 of that Act (duty of authorities to exercise functions under Part III of that Act in accordance with regulations) shall cease to have effect.

(7) Section 36 of that Act (default powers of Minister) shall cease to have effect.

(8) Section 54 of that Act (which enables inquiries to be held for the purposes of that Act) shall cease to have effect.

(9) In paragraph (f) of section 65 of that Act (application to Scotland)—

(a) the words "Part IV of" shall cease to have effect;

(b) at the end there shall be inserted "or section 7 (functions of local authorities) of the Mental Health (Scotland) Act 1984,".

The Public Records Act 1958

6. In Schedule 1 to the Public Records Act 1958 (definition of public records), in the Table in Part I, in the entry relating to the Department of Health, in the second column—

1958 c. 51.

(a) after the words "National Health Service Authorities" there shall be inserted "including National Health Service trusts"; and

(b) for the words "National health service hospitals" there shall be substituted "health service hospitals, within the meaning of the National Health Service Act 1977".

SCH. 9

The Human Tissue Act 1961

1961 c. 54.

7. In section 1 of the Human Tissue Act 1961 (removal of parts of bodies for medical purposes)—

(a) in subsection (4A)(b) after the words "health authority" there shall be inserted "or NHS trust"; and

(b) at the end of subsection (10) there shall be added "and "NHS trust" means a National Health Service trust established under the National Health Service and Community Care Act 1990 or the National Health Service (Scotland) Act 1978".

The Abortion Act 1967

1967 c. 87.

8. In section 1 of the Abortion Act 1967 (medical termination of pregnancy), in subsection (3) after the words "National Health Service (Scotland) Act 1978" there shall be inserted "or in a hospital vested in a National Health Service trust".

The Leasehold Reform Act 1967

1967 c. 88.

9. In section 28 of the Leasehold Reform Act 1967 (retention or resumption of land required for public purposes)—

(a) in subsection (5)(d) for the words "and any special health authority" there shall be substituted "any special health authority and any National Health Service trust"; and

(b) in subsection (6)(c) for the words "or special health authority" there shall be substituted "special health authority or National Health Service trust".

The Social Work (Scotland) Act 1968

1968 c. 49.

10.—(1) The Social Work (Scotland) Act 1968 shall be amended as follows.

(2) In section 2 (the social work committee), in subsection (2) after paragraph (k) there shall be inserted—

"(l) sections 21 to 23 of the Health and Social Services and Social Security Adjudications Act 1983;

(m) the Access to Personal Files Act 1987."

(3) In section 4 (provisions relating to performance of functions by local authorities), after the word "Act", there shall be inserted the words "or section 7 (functions of local authorities) or 8 (provision of after-care services) of the Mental Health (Scotland) Act 1984,".

(4) In section 6 (supervision of establishments), in—

(a) subsection (1)—

(i) for the words "duly authorised officer of", there shall be substituted the words "person duly authorised by"; and

(ii) after the words "of this Act", where they first occur, there shall be inserted the words "or section 7 (functions of local authorities) or 8 (provision of after-care services) of the Mental Health (Scotland) Act 1984";

(b) subsection (1)(a), at the end there shall be inserted ""or section 7 or 8 of the said Act of 1984,";

(c) subsection (2)—

(i) for the word "officer" there shall be substituted the word "person"; and

(ii) after the words "of this Act" there shall be inserted the words "or section 7 or 8 of the said Act of 1984";

(d) subsection (3), for the word "officer" there shall be substituted the words "authorised person"; and

(e) subsection (4), for the words "An officer" there shall be substituted the words "A person".

(5) In section 12 (general social welfare services of local authorities) at the end there shall be inserted—

"(6) For the purposes of subsection (2) of this section 'person in need' includes a person who is in need of care and attention arising out of drug or alcohol dependency or release from prison or other form of detention."

(6) In section 14 (home help), for the words—

(a) "home help", where they first occur there shall be substituted the words "domiciliary services";

(b) "help is", there shall be substituted the words "services are"; and

(c) "home help is", there shall be substituted the words "domiciliary services are".

(7) In section 59(1) (provision of residential and other establishments), at the beginning there shall be inserted the words "Subject to section 13A of this Act,".

(8) In section 61(1A) (definition of "establishment")—

(a) after the word "include" there shall be inserted "(a)"; and

(b) at the end of the definition of "establishment" there shall be inserted—

"; or

(b) any establishment providing residential accommodation with nursing falling within section 13A of this Act;".

(9) In subsection (1) of section 67 (inspection of establishments by local authorities)—

(a) for the words "duly authorised officer of" there shall be substituted the words "person duly authorised by";

(b) for the words "required to be kept therein by virtue of this Part of this Act" there shall be substituted the words "(in whatever form they are held) relating to the place or to any person for whom services have been or are provided there by virtue of this Act or section 7 (functions of local authorities) or 8 (provision of after-care services) of the Mental Health (Scotland) Act 1984";

(c) after the words "subsections (2)", there shall be inserted the words "to (2D)";

(d) for the words "an officer", where they first occur, there shall be substituted the words "a person"; and

(e) for the words "an officer of" there shall be substituted the words "a person authorised by".

(10) In subsection (2) of the said section 67, for the word "officer", in both places where it occurs, there shall be substituted the word "person".

(11) In subsection (1)(d) of section 86 (adjustments between authority providing accommodation etc., and authority of area of residence), at the end there shall be inserted—

"or

(e) in the provision of accommodation, services or facilities for persons ordinarily so resident under section 7 (functions of local authorities) or 8 (provision of after-care services) of the Mental Health (Scotland) Act 1984;".

SCH. 9

(12) In subsection (3) of the said section 86, after the words "1978" there shall be inserted the words "or in a hospital managed by a National Health Service trust established under Part I of the National Health Service and Community Care Act 1990 or section 12A of the National Health Service (Scotland) Act 1978".

(13) In section 87 (charges for services and accommodation),—

(a) in subsection (1), after the words "under this Act", there shall be inserted the words "or section 7 (functions of local authorities) or 8 (provision of after-care services) of the Mental Health (Scotland) Act 1984";

(b) in subsection (1A), after the words "under this Act", there shall be inserted the words "or section 7 or 8 of the said Act of 1984";

(c) in subsections (2), (3) and (4), after the words "under this Act", there shall be inserted the words "or section 7 of the said Act of 1984; and

(d) in subsection (4), after the word "organisation" there shall be inserted the words "or any other person or body".

(14) In subsection (1) of section 94 (interpretation),—

(a) after the definition of "contributor" there shall be inserted the following definition—

""domiciliary services" means any services, being services provided in the home, which appear to a local authority to be necessary for the purpose of enabling a person to maintain as independent an existence as is practicable in his home;"; and

(b) in the definition of "hospital", after the words "1978" there shall be inserted—

"(aa) any hospital managed by a National Health Service trust established under section 12A of the National Health Service (Scotland) Act 1978;".

The Local Authority Social Services Act 1970

1970 c. 42.

11. In Schedule 1 to the Local Authority Social Services Act 1970 (enactments conferring functions assigned to social services committee)—

(a) in the entry relating to the Children Act 1989, in the second column after the words "health authorities" there shall be inserted "National Health Service trusts";

(b) for the entry relating to section 6 of the Local Authority Social Services Act 1970 there shall be substituted—

"Sections 6 and 7B of this Act	Appointment of director of social services, etc; provision and conduct of complaints procedure."; and

(c) at the end of that Schedule there shall be inserted—

"National Health Service and Community Care Act 1990 (c.19)	
Section 46	Preparation of plans for community care services.
Section 47	Assessment of needs for community care services."

The Chronically Sick and Disabled Persons Act 1970

1970 c. 44.

12. In section 2(1) of the Chronically Sick and Disabled Persons Act 1970, the words from "to the provisions" in the first place where they occur, to "the purpose) and" shall be omitted and after the words "Secretary of State)" there shall be inserted "and to the provisions of section 7A of that Act (which requires local authorities to exercise their social services functions in accordance with directions given by the Secretary of State)".

The Local Government Act 1972

1972 c. 70.

13. In section 113 of the Local Government Act 1972 (placing of staff at disposal of other bodies),—

(a) in subsection (1A) after the words "special health authority", in each place where they occur, there shall be inserted "or NHS trust"; and

(b) at the end there shall be added the following subsection—

"(4) In subsection (2A) above "NHS trust" means a National Health Service trust established under Part I of the National Health Service and Community Care Act 1990."

The Criminal Procedure (Scotland) Act 1975

1975 c. 21.

14. In section 462 (interpretation) of the Criminal Procedure (Scotland) Act 1975, in paragraph (a) of the definition of "hospital", after the words "Secretary of State" there shall be inserted the words "or in a National Health Service trust".

The Child Benefit Act 1975

1975 c. 61.

15. In section 3 of the Child Benefit Act 1975 (meaning of "person responsible for child") in subsection (3) (certain days of absence disregarded) in paragraph (c) for the words following "under" there shall be substituted "section 21 of the National Assistance Act 1948, the Children Act 1989 or the Social Work (Scotland) Act 1968."

The Children Act 1975

1975 c. 72.

16. In section 99(1)(b) of the Children Act 1975 (inquiries in Scotland) the words "paragraph (a) of section 1(4) and" shall cease to have effect and after the word "(h)" there shall be inserted "to (k)".

The Adoption Act 1976

17. In section 2 of the Adoption Act 1976 (local authorities' social services) in paragraph (a) (as set out in paragraph 1 of Schedule 10 to the Children Act 1989) after the words "health authorities" there shall be inserted "National Health Service trusts".

The National Health Service Act 1977

1977 c. 49.

18.—(1) In section 41 of the National Health Service Act 1977 (arrangements for pharmaceutical services)—

(a) for the words "supply to persons who are in that locality" there shall be substituted "provision to persons who are in that locality of";

(b) in paragraph (b) after the words "health authority" there shall be inserted "or an NHS trust" and the word "and" at the end of the paragraph shall be omitted; and

(c) after paragraph (c) there shall be inserted "and

(d) such other services as may be prescribed."

SCH. 9

(2) At the end of section 43 of that Act (persons authorised to provide pharmaceutical services) there shall be added the following subsection—

"(3) No arrangements for the provision of pharmaceutical services falling within section 41(d) above shall be made with persons other than those who are registered pharmacists or are of a prescribed description."

(3) In section 63 of that Act (hospital accommodation on part payment) after subsection (1) there shall be inserted the following subsection—

"(1C) References in subsection (1) above to a health service hospital do not include references to a hospital vested in an NHS trust."

(4) At the end of section 65 of that Act (accommodation and services for private patients) there shall be added the following subsection—

"(4) References in the preceding provisions of this section to a health service hospital do not include references to a hospital vested in an NHS trust."

(5) In section 83A of that Act (remission and repayment of charges and payment of travelling expenses) in subsection (1)—

(a) in paragraph (b) after the words "Secretary of State" there shall be inserted "or an NHS trust" and at the end there shall be added "and", and

(b) after paragraph (b) there shall be inserted the following paragraph—

"(c) for the reimbursement by a District Health Authority to an NHS trust and, in such cases as may be prescribed to another District Health Authority, of payments made by virtue of exercising the functions conferred under paragraph (b) above".

(6) In section 84 of that Act (inquiries) at the end of subsection (1) there shall be added the words "or Part I of the National Health Service and Community Care Act 1990".

(7) In section 85 of that Act (default powers)—

(a) in subsection (1), for paragraph (e) there shall be substituted the following paragraph—

"(e) an NHS trust";

and in the words following paragraph (g) after the words "this Act" there shall be inserted "or Part I of the National Health Service and Community Care Act 1990";

(b) in subsection (2), for the words from the beginning to "body shall" there shall be substituted "The members of the body in default shall";

(c) subsections (3) and (4) shall be omitted.

(8) In section 86 of that Act (emergency powers) after the words "this Act", in the first place where they occur, there shall be inserted "or Part I of the National Health Service and Community Care Act 1990" and after the words "this Act", in the second place where they occur, there shall be inserted "or that Part".

(9) At the end of section 103 of that Act (special arrangement as to payment of remuneration) there shall be inserted the following subsection—

"(3) If the Secretary of State by order so provides with respect to remuneration in respect of such pharmaceutical services as may be specified in the order,—

(a) an NHS trust determined in accordance with the order shall have the function of paying sums so determined to the Family Health Services Authority which, under Part II of this Act, has the function of paying that remuneration; and

SCH. 9

(b) nothing in subsection (2) above shall apply with respect to that remuneration."

(10) In section 109 of that Act, after paragraph (d) there shall be inserted—

"(da) NHS trusts".

(11) In section 110 of that Act (investigations for England and for Wales), after paragraph (b) there shall be inserted—

"(ba) an NHS trust which is managing a hospital or other establishment or facility which is in Wales".

(12) In section 122 of that Act (recovery of charges), in subsection (1) after the words "this Act", in the second place where they occur, there shall be inserted "or Part I of the National Health Service and Community Care Act 1990".

(13) In Schedule 7 to that Act (additional provisions as to Community Health Councils), in paragraph 2—

(a) in sub-paragraph (d) after the word "by" there shall be inserted "Regional Health Authorities, NHS trusts"; and

(b) in sub-paragraph (e) for the words from "such Authorities", in the first place where those words appear, to the end of the sub-paragraph there shall be inserted "Regional and District Health Authorities, NHS trusts or relevant Family Health Services Authorities, and the right of members of Councils to enter and inspect premises controlled by such health authorities or NHS trusts".

(14) In Schedule 8 to that Act (local social services authorities' functions)—

(a) in paragraph 1 (care of mothers) after the word "mothers" there shall be inserted "(other than for the provision of residential accommodation for them)";

(b) in paragraph 2 (prevention, care and after-care)—

(i) sub-paragraphs (1)(a) and (4) (which make provision respectively for the provision by authorities of residential accommodation and for regulations to be made conferring powers of inspection of certain premises provided under that paragraph) shall cease to have effect; and

(ii) after sub-paragraph (4A) there shall be inserted—

"(4AA) No authority is authorised or may be required under this paragraph to provide residential accommodation for any person."

The National Health Service (Scotland) Act 1978

19.—(1) In section 2 of the National Health Service (Scotland) Act 1978 (Health Boards), in subsection (5) after the words "subsection (1)" there shall be inserted "and in exercising any function otherwise conferred on them by or under this Act".

1978 c. 29.

(2) In subsection (5) of section 11 (Scottish Hospital Trust) of that Act, after the words "and shall cause" there shall be inserted the words "such accounts to be audited and".

(3) In section 12 of that Act (Scottish Hospital Endowments Research Trust), after subsection (4) there shall be inserted the following subsections—

"(4A) The Research Trust shall have power to engage in activities intended to stimulate the giving of money or other property to assist them in carrying out the purpose aforesaid.

(4B) Subject to any directions of the Secretary of State excluding specified activities or descriptions of activity, the activities authorised by subsection (4A) include public appeals or collections, and the soliciting of sponsorship, donations, legacies, bequests and gifts."

SCH. 9

(4) In section 13 of that Act (co-operation between Health Boards and other authorities), after the word "Boards," there shall be inserted "NHS trusts,".

(5) In subsection (1)(a) of section 13A of that Act (co-operation in planning of services for disabled persons, the elderly and others) for the words from "being" to the end there shall be substituted the words "by Health Boards and such of the authorities mentioned in that section as may be concerned;".

(6) For paragraph (b) of subsection (2) of section 25 of that Act (arrangements for provision of general dental services) there shall be substituted the following paragraph—

"(b) for conferring a right, subject to—

(i) subsection (2A);

(ii) the provisions of this Part relating to the disqualification of persons providing services; and

(iii) section 8 (persons over retiring age) of the Health and Medicines Act 1988 and regulations made under that section,

on any dental practitioner who wishes to be included in any such list to be so included;".

(7) In section 27 of that Act (arrangements for provision of pharmaceutical services)—

(a) in subsection (1)—

(i) for the word "supply" there shall be substituted "provision";

(ii) in paragraph (b), after the word "Board" there shall be inserted "or by an NHS trust";

(iii) at the end of paragraph (c) there shall be inserted—

"; and

(d) such services as may be prescribed,"; and

(iv) for the words "services provided in accordance with the arrangements are" there shall be substituted "provision of drugs, medicines, appliances and services in accordance with the arrangements is";

(b) in subsection (2), after the word "mentioned" in the second place where it occurs there shall be inserted ", or to whom services mentioned in subsection (1)(d) are to be provided,";

(c) in subsections (3)(b), (c) and (d) and (4), before the word "services" in each place where it occurs there shall be inserted "pharmaceutical"; and

(d) in subsection (4)(d) for the words "a prescribed criterion" there shall be substituted "prescribed criteria".

(8) In section 28(2) of that Act (persons authorised to provide pharmaceutical services)—

(a) after the word "medicines" in the first place where it occurs there shall be inserted "or the provision of pharmaceutical services";

(b) after the word "undertake" there shall be inserted "(a)";

(c) for the word "supplied" there shall be substituted "provided"; and

(d) after the word "dispensed" there shall be inserted—

", and

(b) that all services mentioned in section 27(1)(d) provided by them under those arrangements shall be provided,".

(9) In section 55(1) (hospital accommodation on part payment) of that Act, after the word "hospital" there shall be inserted the words "vested in the Secretary of State".

SCH. 9

(10) In section 57(1) (accommodation and services for private patients), after the word "hospital" where it first occurs there shall be inserted "vested in the Secretary of State".

(11) In section 73 of that Act (charges for more expensive supplies) at the end there shall be inserted—

"(c) by a National Health Service trust in respect of the supply by them of any appliance or vehicle which is, at the request of the person supplied, of a more expensive type than the prescribed type, or in respect of the replacement or repair of any such appliance, or the replacement of any such vehicle.".

(12) In section 74 of that Act (charges for repairs and replacement in certain cases), after paragraph (b) there shall be inserted—

"or

(c) by an NHS trust in respect of the replacement or repair of any appliance or vehicle supplied by them,".

(13) In section 75A of that Act (remission and repayment of charges and payment of travelling expenses)—

(a) in subsection (1), at the end there shall be inserted—

"and

(d) for the payment by the Secretary of State to NHS trusts of such sums as will reimburse them for any sums paid by them as travelling expenses in such cases as may be prescribed"; and

(b) in subsection (2), for the words "or (c)" there shall be substituted the words ", (c) or (d)".

(14) In section 77 of that Act (default powers), after paragraph (a) of subsection (1) there shall be inserted—

"(aa) an NHS trust".

(15) In section 79 of that Act (purchase of land and moveable property)—

(a) in subsection (1), after the word "Act" where it first appears there shall be inserted the words "and may take any such property or land on lease,"; and

(b) in subsection (2), after the word "(1)," there shall be inserted the words "other than on lease".

(16) In section 84 of that Act (power of trustees to make payments to Health Boards)—

(a) in subsection (1), after the words "Health Board" where they—

(i) second occur, there shall be inserted the words "or an NHS trust"; and

(ii) third occur, there shall be inserted the words "or NHS trust";

(b) in subsection (2)—

(i) after the words "Health Board" there shall be inserted the words "or NHS trust"; and

(ii) after the word "Boards" there shall be inserted the words "or NHS trusts". and

(c) in subsection (3), after the words "Health Board" there shall be inserted the words "or an NHS trust".

(17) In section 84A of that Act (power to raise money by appeals etc)—

(a) in subsection (1), after the word "Board" there shall be inserted "or NHS trust"; and

SCH. 9

(b) in subsections (3) to (7), after the word "Board" in each place where it occurs there shall be inserted ", NHS trust".

(18) In section 93(1) of that Act (bodies subject to investigation by Health Service Commissioner for Scotland), after paragraph (b) there shall be inserted—

"(bb) NHS trusts".

(19) In section 101 of that Act (protection of health bodies and their officers), after the word "Board" there shall be inserted ", an NHS trust".

(20) In section 102(1) of that Act (management of state hospitals), for the word "90(2)" there shall be substituted "91(2)".

(21) In section 105 of that Act (orders, regulations and directions)—

(a) after subsection (1) there shall be inserted the following subsection—

"(1A) Subsection (1) does not apply to orders made under section 12D(1) or paragraph 26(1) of Schedule 7A.";

(b) in subsection (4), after the words "10(3) to (5)" there shall be inserted the words "12A(1), 12A(8), 12E(1), 12G(2),"; and

(c) at the end of the said subsection (4) there shall be inserted the words "paragraph 25(1) of Schedule 7A and paragraph 3 of Schedule 7B".

(22) In section 108(1) of that Act (interpretation)—

(a) in the definition of "Health Board", for the word "board" there shall be substituted the words "Health Board";

(b) at the end of the definition of "health service hospital" there shall be added "or vested in an NHS trust";

(c) after the definition of "modifications" there shall be inserted—

""National Health Service trust" has the meaning indicated by section 12A and "NHS trust" shall be construed accordingly"; and

"NHS contract" has the meaning indicated by section 17A(3)";

(d) after the definition of "officer" there shall be inserted—

"'operational date", in relation to an NHS trust, shall be construed in accordance with paragraph 3(1)(e) of Schedule 7A;"; and

(e) after the definition of "the Research Trust" there shall be inserted—

""Special Health Board" means a Special Health Board constituted under section 2;".

(23) In section 110 of that Act (citation, extent and commencement)—

(a) in subsection (2), for the words "subsection (3)" there shall be substituted "subsections (2A) and (3)"; and

(b) after subsection (2) there shall be inserted—

"(2A) Section 87B(3) extends also to England and Wales."

(24) In Schedule 6 to that Act (the Hospital Trust)—

(a) in paragraph 4(c), after the words "Health Boards" there shall be inserted the words "and NHS trusts";

(b) after paragraph 4(e) there shall be inserted—

"(ea) power to accept from any NHS trust for investment and management on behalf of the trust any property held on behalf of the trust by trustees appointed by virtue of section 12G(2), and any endowments or accumulated income otherwise held by the trust;";

(c) in paragraph 4(f)—

(i) after the words "paragraph (e)" there shall be inserted the words "or, as the case may be, paragraph (ea)"; and

(ii) after the words "Health Board" there shall be inserted the words "or, as the case may be, by an NHS Trust";

(d) in paragraph 6(2), after the words "Health Boards" there shall be inserted the words "or NHS trusts";

(e) in paragraph 7(1), after the words "Health Boards" there shall be inserted the words ", NHS trusts";

(f) in paragraph 7(2), after the words "Health Boards" there shall be inserted the words ", NHS trusts"; and

(g) in paragraph 7(3), at the end there shall be inserted—

"(c) in so far as it is distributed among NHS trusts, being used by that trust for any purpose for which the trust was established."

The Employment Protection (Consolidation) Act 1978

1978 c. 44.

20. In the Employment Protection (Consolidation) Act 1978, in section 29 (time off for public duties) in subsection (1)(d) after the words "member of" there shall be inserted "a National Health Service trust or".

The Overseas Development and Co-operation Act 1980

1980 c. 63.

21. In the Overseas Development and Co-operation Act 1980, in Schedule 1 (statutory bodies with powers under section 2(1))—

(a) in Part II, in the heading, after the words "NATIONAL HEALTH SERVICE ACT 1977" there shall be inserted "AND THE NATIONAL HEALTH SERVICE AND COMMUNITY CARE ACT 1990";

(b) at the end of that Part there shall be inserted "National Health Service trusts"; and

(c) at the end of Part IV (bodies constituted under the National Health Service (Scotland) Act 1978), there shall be inserted "National Health Service trusts".

The Education Act 1981

1981 c. 60.

22. In the Education Act 1981, in section 10 (duty of health authority to notify parents)—

(a) in subsection (1), after the words "Health Authority" there shall be inserted "or a National Health Service trust"; and

(b) after the words "the Authority", in each place where they appear, there shall be inserted "or trust".

The Acquisition of Land Act 1981

1981 c. 67.

23. In the Acquisition of Land Act 1981, in section 17 (local authority and statutory undertakers' land), in subsection (4), in the definition of "statutory undertakers" after paragraph (a) there shall be inserted—

"(aa) a National Health Service trust established under Part I of the National Health Service and Community Care Act 1990, and".

The Mental Health Act 1983

1983 c. 20.

24.—(1) In section 12 of the Mental Health Act 1983 (general provisions as to medical recommendations), in subsection (3) after the words "National Health Service Act 1977" there shall be inserted "or paragraph 14 of Schedule 2 to the National Health Service and Community Care Act 1990".

SCH. 9

(2) In section 19 of that Act (regulations as to transfer of patients), in subsection (3)—

(a) after the words "such a hospital" there shall be inserted "or in a hospital vested in a National Health Service trust", and

(b) for the words from "for which the managers" to "also the managers", there shall be substituted "which is managed by the managers of, or is vested in the National Health Service trust for, the first-mentioned hospital".

(3) In section 23 of that Act (discharge of patients)—

(a) in subsection (3) after the words "a contract with a" there shall be inserted "National Health Service trust", and after the words "by that" there shall be inserted "trust or", and

(b) in subsection (4), after the word "exercised" there shall be inserted "subject to subsection (5) below" and after the word "authority", in each place in which it occurs, there shall be inserted "trust", and

(c) after subsection (4) there shall be inserted the following subsection—

"(5) The reference in subsection (4) above to the members of an authority, trust or body or the members of a committee or sub-committee of an authority, trust or body,—

(a) in the case of a District or Special Health Authority or a committee or sub-committee of such an authority, is a reference only to the chairman of the authority and such members (of the authority, committee or sub-committee, as the case may be) as are not also officers of the authority, within the meaning of the National Health Service Act 1977; and

(b) in the case of a National Health Service trust or a committee or sub-committee of such a trust, is a reference only to the chairman of the trust and such directors or (in the case of a committee or sub-committee) members as are not also employees of the trust."

(4) In section 24 of that Act (visiting and examination of patients), in subsection (3) after the words "District Health Authority" there shall be inserted "National Health Service trust"; and in paragraph (a) of that subsection after the word "authority" there shall be inserted "or trust".

(5) In section 32 of that Act (regulations for purposes of Part II), in subsection (3) after the words "District Health Authorities" there shall be inserted "National Health Service trusts" and for the words "and authorities" there shall be inserted "authorities and trusts".

(6) In section 117 of that Act (after-care) in subsection (3) for the words "the District Health Authority for the district" there shall be substituted "such District Health Authority as may be determined in accordance with regulations made by the Secretary of State".

(7) In section 139 of that Act (protection for acts done in pursuance of the Act), at the end of subsection (4) there shall be inserted "or against a National Health Service trust established under the National Health Service and Community Care Act 1990".

(8) In section 140 of that Act (notification of hospitals having arrangements for reception of urgent cases) after the words "administered by" there shall be inserted "or otherwise available to".

(9) In section 145(1) of that Act (definitions) in the definition of "the managers", after paragraph (b) there shall be inserted the following paragraph—

"(bb) in relation to a hospital vested in a National Health Service trust, the directors of the trust".

The Health and Social Services and Social Security Adjudications Act 1983

SCH. 9

1983 c. 41.

25.—(1) In section 17 of the Health and Social Services and Social Security Adjudications Act 1983 (charges for local authority services in England and Wales) after paragraph (e) of subsection (2) (services to which that section applies) there shall be inserted "other than the provision of services for which payment may be required under section 22 or 26 of the National Assistance Act 1948".

(2) In subsection (8) of section 21 of that Act (recovery of sums due to local authority where persons in residential accommodation have disposed of assets), at the end there shall be inserted the words "or section 7 (functions of local authorities) of the Mental Health (Scotland) Act 1984,".

The Public Health (Control of Disease) Act 1984

1984 c. 22.

26.—(1) In section 13 of the Public Health (Control of Disease) Act 1984 (regulations for control of certain diseases), in subsection (4), in paragraph (a) after the words "District Health Authorities" there shall be inserted "National Health Service trusts".

(2) In section 37 of that Act (removal to hospital of person with notifiable disease), in subsection (1)—

(a) in paragraph (c) after the words "Secretary of State" there shall be inserted "or, pursuant to arrangements made by a District Health Authority (whether under an NHS contract or otherwise), in a suitable hospital vested in a NHS trust or other person"; and

(b) in the words following paragraph (c) for the words from "responsible" to "the hospital" there shall be substituted "in whose district lies the area, or the greater part of the area, of the local authority".

(3) In section 41 of that Act (removal to hospital of inmate of common lodging-house with notifiable disease), in subsection (1)—

(a) in paragraph (c) after the words "Secretary of State" there shall be inserted "or, pursuant to arrangements made by a District Health Authority (whether under an NHS contract or otherwise) in a suitable hospital vested in an NHS trust or any other person"; and

(b) in the words following paragraph (c) for the words from "responsible" to "of the hospital" there shall be substituted "in whose district lies the area, or the greater part of the area, of the local authority".

(4) In section 74 of that Act(definitions) after the definition of "London port health authority" there shall be inserted—

""NHS trust" and "NHS contract" have the same meaning as in Part I of the National Health Service and Community Care Act 1990 or, as the case may require, the National Health Service (Scotland) Act 1978".

The Registered Homes Act 1984

1984 c. 23.

27. In section 21 of the Registered Homes Act 1984 (meaning of "nursing home") in subsection (3)(a) (premises excluded from the definition) for the words "hospital or" there shall be substituted "health service hospital, within the meaning of the National Health Service Act 1977, or any".

The Mental Health (Scotland) Act 1984

1984 c. 36.

28.—(1) In subsection (2)(e) of section 3 (functions and duties of the Mental Welfare Commission) of the Mental Health (Scotland) Act 1984 after the words "Health Board"—

(a) where they first occur, there shall be inserted the words ", a National Health Service trust established under section 12A of the National Health Service (Scotland) Act 1978"; and

SCH. 9

(b) where they second occur, there shall be inserted the words ", the National Health Service trust".

(2) In subsection (2)(a) of section 12 (registration of private hospitals) of that Act, after the words "Secretary of State" there shall be inserted the words "or managed by a National Health Service trust established under section 12A of the National Health Service (Scotland) Act 1978."

(3) In section 20(1)(c) (medical recommendations: hospital) of that Act—

(a) for the words "or 58 of" there shall be substituted the words "of, or paragraph 14 of Schedule 7A to,"; and

(b) for the word "relates" there shall be substituted the word "relate".

(4) In subsection (1) of section 125 (interpretation) of that Act—

(a) in the definition of "hospital", after paragraph (a) there shall be inserted—

"(aa) any hospital managed by a National Health Service trust established under section 12A of the said Act of 1978;";

(b) in the definition of "managers of a hospital", after paragraph (a) there shall be inserted—

"(aa) in relation to a hospital managed by a National Health Service trust established under section 12A (National Health Service trusts) of the said Act of 1978, the directors of the trust;".

The Hospital Complaints Procedure Act 1985

1985 c. 42.

29. After section 1 of the Hospital Complaints Procedure Act 1985 there shall be inserted—

"1A. It shall also be the duty of the Secretary of State to give directions under paragraph 6(2)(e) of Schedule 2 to the National Health Service and Community Care Act 1990 and paragraph 6(2)(e) of Schedule 7A to the National Health Service (Scotland) Act 1978, to any NHS trust which is responsible for the management of a hospital, to comply with directions under section 1 above."

The Disabled Persons (Services, Consultation and Representation) Act 1986

1986 c. 33.

30.—(1) In section 2 of the Disabled Persons (Services, Consultation and Representation) Act 1986 (rights of authorised representatives of disabled persons), in subsection (5) (by virtue of which a disabled person's authorised representative may visit and interview him in various categories of accommodation)—

(a) in paragraph (a) (hospital accommodation) after the words "the 1977 Act" there shall be inserted "or by a National Health Service trust established under the provisions of the National Health Service and Community Care Act 1990" and after the words "the 1978 Act" there shall be inserted "or by a National Health Service trust established under that Act";

(b) in paragraph (c) (accommodation provided by a voluntary organisation in accordance with arrangements made under section 26 of the National Assistance Act 1948) after the word "organisation", in the first place where it occurs, there shall be inserted the words "or other person"; and

1989 c. 41.

(c) in paragraph (cc) (which is inserted by paragraph 59(4) of Schedule 13 to the Children Act 1989) after the word "organisation" there shall be inserted the words "or other person".

(2) In section 7 of that Act (persons discharged from hospital), in subsection (9), in the definition of "managers" the word "and" at the end of paragraph (c) shall be omitted and after that paragraph there shall be inserted—

"(cc) in relation to a hospital vested in a National Health Service trust means the directors of that trust; and".

The Education (No. 2) Act 1986

1986 c. 61.

31. In section 7 of the Education (No. 2) Act 1986 (appointment of representative governors) in subsection (2), for the words following "provide" there shall be substituted—

"(a) in the case of a hospital vested in the Secretary of State, for one governor to be appointed by the District Health Authority; and

(b) in the case of a hospital vested in a National Health Service trust, for one governor to be appointed by that trust."

The AIDS (Control) Act 1987

1987 c. 33.

32.—(1) Section 1 of the AIDS (Control) Act 1987 (periodical reports on matters relating to AIDS and HIV) shall be amended as follows—

(a) in subsection (1), in paragraph (b) the word "and" at the end of sub-paragraph (ii) shall be deleted and at the end of sub-paragraph (iii) there shall be inserted—

"and
(iv) each NHS trust";

(b) in subsection (2) after the words "District Health Authority" in the first place where they occur, there shall be inserted "an NHS trust";

(c) in subsection (3) after the words "District Health Authority" there shall be inserted "NHS trust" and after the words "by the Authority" there shall be inserted "trust"; and

(d) at the end there shall be added—

"(10) In this section "NHS trust" means a National Health Service trust established under Part I of the National Health Service and Community Care Act 1990 or, as the case may be, under the National Health Service (Scotland) Act 1978."

(2) In the Schedule to that Act (contents of reports), after the word "Authority", in each place in which that word appears, there shall be inserted "NHS trust".

The Community Health Councils (Access to Information) Act 1988

1988 c. 24.

33. In section 1 of the Community Health Councils (Access to Information) Act 1988 (access to meetings and documents of Community Health Councils), in subsection (6)(a) after the words "exercises functions" there shall be inserted "or any National Health Service trust which is established under Part I of the National Health Service and Community Care Act 1990 and carries on any of its activities from premises in the area of the authority".

The Health and Medicines Act 1988

1988 c. 49.

34. In section 7 of the Health and Medicines Act 1988 (extension of powers for financing the health service) in subsection (2), after the word "powers", in the second place where it occurs, there shall be inserted "(exercisable outside as well as within Great Britain)".

SCH. 9

The Road Traffic Act 1988

1988 c. 52.

35. In section 161 of the Road Traffic Act 1988 (interpretation) in subsection (1), in the definition of "hospital" for the word "an", in the first place where it occurs, there shall be substituted "any health service hospital, within the meaning of the National Health Service Act 1977 or the National Health Service (Scotland) Act 1978 and any other".

The Children Act 1989

1989 c. 41.

36.—(1) In section 21 of the Children Act 1989 (provision of accommodation for children in police protection etc.), in subsection (3) after the words "vested in the Secretary of State" shall be inserted the words "or otherwise made available pursuant to arrangements made by a District Health Authority".

(2) In section 24 of that Act (advice and assistance for certain children)—

(a) at the end of subsection (2)(d)(ii) there shall be added the words "or in any accommodation provided by a National Health Service trust"; and

(b) at the end of subsection (12)(c) there shall be added the words "or any accommodation provided by a National Health Service trust".

(3) In section 29 of that Act (recoupment of cost of providing services etc.), at the end of paragraph (c) of subsection (8) there shall be added the words "or any other hospital made available pursuant to arrangements made by a District Health Authority".

(4) In section 80 of that Act (inspection of children's homes etc.).—

(a) in subsection (1)(d) after the words "health authority" there shall be inserted "or National Health Service trust"; and

(b) in subsection (5)(e) after the words "health authority" there shall be inserted "National Health Service trust".

(5) In section 85 of that Act (children accommodated by health authorities and local education authorities), in subsection (1) after the words "health authority" there shall be inserted "National Health Service trust".

The Opticians Act 1989

1989 c. 44.

37. In section 27 of the Opticians Act 1989 (sale and supply of optical appliances), at the end of subsection (4)(b)(i) there shall be inserted "or the National Health Service and Community Care Act 1990".

Section 66(2).

SCHEDULE 10

ENACTMENTS REPEALED

Chapter	Short title	Extent of repeal
1 & 2 Geo. 6 c. 73.	The Nursing Homes Registration (Scotland) Act 1938.	Section 1(3)(bb) and (bc).
11 & 12 Geo. 6 c. 29.	The National Assistance Act 1948.	In section 21(8) the words from the beginning to "subsection". Section 22(7). In section 26, in subsections (2) and (5) the words "subsection (1) of". Section 35(2) and (3). Section 36.

SCH. 10

Chapter	Short title	Extent of repeal
		In section 41(1) the words "the Mental Health Act 1959, or". Section 54.
7 & 8 Eliz.2 c. 72.	The Mental Health Act 1959.	In section 8, subsection (1), in subsection (2) the words from the beginning to "description; and" and the words "accommodation or" in the second place where they occur and subsection (3).
1968 c. 46.	The Health Services and Public Health Act 1968.	Section 44(1). In section 45, in subsection (5), in paragraph (b) the word "36" and in paragraph (c) the word "54".
1968 c. 49.	The Social Work (Scotland) Act 1968.	In section 1, in subsection (4)(b), the word "and", and subsection (4)(c).
1970 c. 44.	The Chronically Sick and Disabled Persons Act 1970.	In section 2(1) the words from "to the provisions" in the first place where they occur, to "the purpose) and".
1971 c. 40.	The Fire Precautions Act 1971.	In section 40, subsections (2)(c) and (10).
1972 c. 70.	The Local Government Act 1972.	In Schedule 23, in paragraph 2, in sub-paragraph (3) the words from "in subsection (1)" to "whereby" and" and "of that section" and sub-paragraph (7), and paragraph 9(1).
1973 c. 32.	The National Health Service Reorganisation Act 1973.	In Schedule 4, paragraph 45.
1975 c. 14.	The Social Security Act 1975.	In section 35(6)(a) the words from "paragraph 2" to "1977".
1975 c. 22.	The Children Act 1975.	In section 99(1)(b) the words "paragraph (a) of section 1(4) and".
1976 c. 83.	The Health Services Act 1976.	The whole Act.

SCH. 10

Chapter	Short title	Extent of repeal
1977 c. 49.	The National Health Service Act 1977.	In section 8, in subsection (1) the word "areas", in each place where it occurs, and in paragraph (b) the word "or", where it first appears; subsection (1A)(b); in subsection (2) the words "area or" (and "Area or"), in each place where they occur; in subsection (3) the words "areas or" and "area or"; subsection (5). Section 10(7). In section 11(1) the words "Area or". In section 12(a) the words "Area Health Authorities". In section 13(1) the words "an Area Health Authority of which the area is in Wales". In section 14 the words "Area or" and "area or", in each place where they occur. In section 16, in subsection (1) the words "Area or", where they occur in paragraphs (c) and (d); in subsection (2) the words "an Area Health Authority", in the first place where they occur, and the words "an Area Health Authority and a District Health Authority are equivalent to each other". In section 18(3) the words "Area or". Section 33(7). In section 41(b) the final word "and". Section 55. Section 85(1)(e), (3) and (4). In section 91(3)(b) the words "Area or". In section 97(6) the word "Area". In section 98, subsections (1)(b) and (3). Section 99(1)(b). In Schedule 5, Parts I and II in paragraph 8 the words "Area Health Authority" and paragraph 15(2).

Chapter	Short title	Extent of repeal
		In Schedule 8, in paragraph 2, sub-paragraph (1)(a), in sub-paragraph (3) the words "residential accommodation or", and sub-paragraph (4). In Schedule 14, in paragraph 13(1)(b) the word "44". In Schedule 15, paragraphs 5, 24(1), 63 and 67.
1978 c. 29.	The National Health Service (Scotland) Act 1978.	Section 2(9). Sections 5 and 6. In section 7(2), the words from "by local authorities" to "and for the appointment". In section 10, in subsection (4), the words "the Planning Council", and subsection (9). Section 13A(1)(c). Section 13B. Section 23(7). Section 57(3). Section 85(1)(a). Section 86(2). In section 108(1), the definitions of "the national consultative committees" and "the Planning Council". Schedule 3. In Schedule 15, in paragraph 10(b) "82" and paragraph 15.
1978 c. 44.	The Employment Protection (Consolidation) Act 1978.	In section 99, in subsection (1), paragraph (c) and the word "or" immediately preceding it. In section 111(1)(a) the words "or paragraph (c)". Section 138(5). Section 149(1)(d). Schedule 5.
1980 c. 53.	The Health Services Act 1980.	Sections 12 to 15. Section 22. In Schedule 1, paragraph 5; in paragraph 78, sub-paragraphs (2) to (6); paragraph 79. In Schedule 2, paragraphs 1 to 6. Schedule 3.

SCH. 10

Chapter	Short title	Extent of repeal
		In Schedule 4, paragraph 7(b).
1983 c. 20.	The Mental Health Act 1983.	Section 124. In section 135(6) the words from "or under" to "1977".
1983 c. 41.	The Health and Social Services and Social Security Adjudications Act 1983.	In section 30, in subsection (3), paragraph (a) and in the words following paragraph (b) the words "2(1) and" and "respectively".
1984 c. 22.	The Public Health (Control of Disease) Act 1984.	In section 37(1) the words "Area or". In section 41(1) the words "Area or".
1984 c. 23.	The Registered Homes Act 1984.	Section 25(1)(d) and (e).
1984 c. 36.	The Mental Health (Scotland) Act 1984.	Section 13(1)(c).
1984 c. 48.	The Health and Social Security Act 1984.	In Schedule 3, paragraphs 6(a) and 12.
1986 c. 33.	The Disabled Persons (Services, Consultation and Representation) Act 1986.	In section 2(5)(b), the words "or Schedule 8 to the 1977 Act".
1986 c. 50.	The Social Security Act 1986.	In Schedule 10, paragraph 32(2).
1986 c. 66.	The National Health Service (Amendment) Act 1986.	Sections 1 and 2.
1988 c. 9.	The Local Government Act 1988.	In Schedule 1, in paragraph 2(4)(b) the words from "Schedule 8" to "1977".
1988 c. 41.	The Local Government Finance Act 1988.	In Schedule 1, in paragraph 9(2)(b) the words from "or paragraph" to "1977".
1988 c. 49.	The Health and Medicines Act 1988.	In Schedule 2, paragraph 11.
1989 c. 42.	The Local Government and Housing Act 1989.	In section 184, subsections (1) and (3).
1990 c. 19.	The National Health Service and Community Care Act 1990.	Section 36(5).

PRINTED IN THE UNITED KINGDOM BY PAUL FREEMAN
Controller and Chief Executive of Her Majesty's Stationery Office
and Queen's Printer of Acts of Parliament
1st Impression July 1990
2nd Impression July 1991